SUPER EASY PLANT-BASED COOKBOOK

SUPER EASY
PLANT-BASED
COOKBOOK

Healthy Recipes for One-Pot, 5-Ingredient, 30-Minute, No-Cook Meals

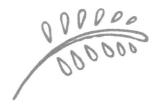

KATHY A. DAVIS

PHOTOGRAPHY BY MARIJA VIDAL

ROCKRIDGE
PRESS

For general information on our other products and services or to obtain technical support, please contact our Customer Care Department within the United States at (866) 744-2665, or outside the United States at (510) 253-0500.

Rockridge Press publishes its books in a variety of electronic and print formats. Some content that appears in print may not be available in electronic books, and vice versa.

TRADEMARKS: Rockridge Press and the Rockridge Press logo are trademarks or registered trademarks of Callisto Media Inc. and/or its affiliates, in the United States and other countries, and may not be used without written permission. All other trademarks are the property of their respective owners. Rockridge Press is not associated with any product or vendor mentioned in this book.

Interior and Cover Designer: Erik Jacobsen
Art Producer: Sue Bischofberger
Editor: Van Van Cleave
Production Editor: Ashley Polikoff
Photography © 2021 Marija Vidal; food styling by Elisabet der Nederlanden

Cover: Rainbow Vegetable Sandwiches, page 43

ISBN: Print 978-1-64876-940-5
eBook 978-1-64876-272-7
R0

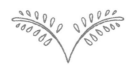

This book is dedicated you, the reader.
I hope this book inspires you to
adopt a plant-focused lifestyle.

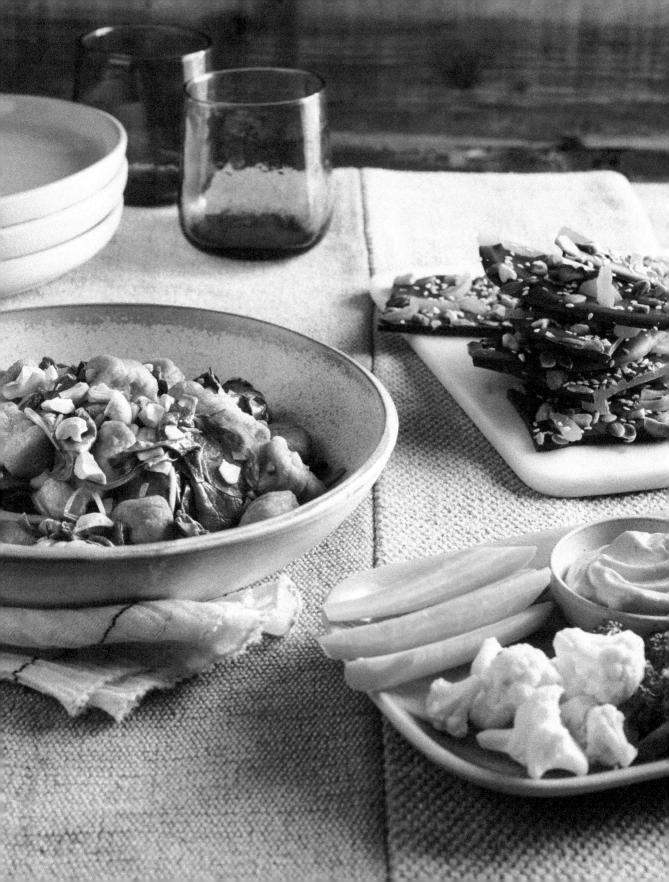

Contents

Chapter 4:

30-MINUTE MEALS   45

Chapter 5:

5-INGREDIENT MEALS   69

Chapter 6:

ONE-POT MEALS 93

Chapter 7:

SUPER EASY SNACKS AND DESSERTS 117

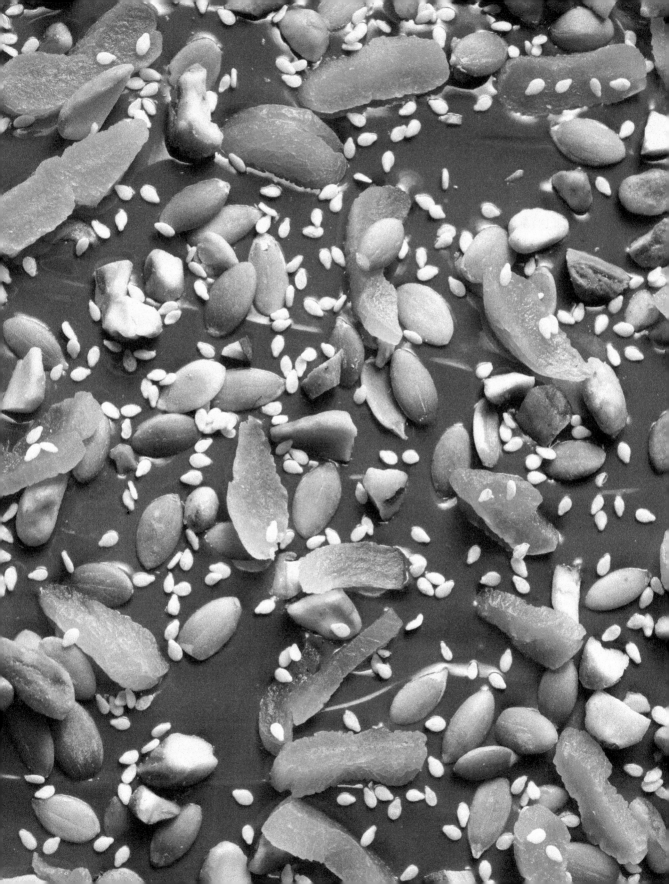

Introduction

By now, you've probably heard the phrase "plant-based diet" and wondered what exactly it means. The phrase seems to be popping up everywhere: we hear it on talk shows, read about it in cooking magazines and blogs, and even see big restaurants chains offering different types of plant-based "fast food." But plant-based diets are more than just trends or buzzwords. They are a real, nourishing, and easy way to eat healthy.

You may think that plant-based eating means learning new and difficult cooking techniques; buying expensive, unfamiliar ingredients you only use a few times; or trying to find time you don't actually have to make complicated dishes. Not so! This book will introduce you to a different type of plant-based diet: quick and healthy meals you can whip up anytime; with minimal, easy-to-find ingredients; in 30 minutes or less. Because, let's face it: between work, school, and errands, most people have fewer than 30 minutes a day to prepare dinner anyway! We want delicious, healthy meals—but fast. It seems even harder for plant-based eaters because certain foods are quite literally off the table. The good news is that more resources than ever are available to make your goal of plant-based eating a reality. This book shows you how to have a plant-based diet that is appetizing and effortless.

My journey started in 2013 after my husband, John, read two contradictory articles about healthy eating in a magazine (one saying animal products were healthy, and one saying animal products contained cholesterol and were unhealthy). This was understandably confusing and led him to do more research. He found articles from plant-based doctors, such as Dr. Caldwell Esselstyn, Dr. T. Colin Campbell, and Dr. John McDougall, about the benefits of plant-based eating, and he shared them with me. We learned that animal products did in fact contain types of cholesterol that could lead to heart-related illnesses. Before that, we had considered our diet—focused on eating organic or locally grown products, including meats, cheeses, produce, etc.—to be healthy, but we were shocked to discover it wasn't as healthy as we thought.

John had always been interested in the science behind health and muscle building (and I just went along with it because he did more of the cooking). But the more plant-based meals I tried and enjoyed, the easier it became for me to leave behind animal products. Every time I tried a new recipe or plant-focused meal, I got excited about how delicious the meal turned out and how little I missed animal products. Using ingredients like avocados for creaminess and squash blended with spices in a cheesy-style sauce left me happy and satisfied.

After about six months of trying new recipes and realizing that a plant-based lifestyle wasn't as restrictive as I believed, I fully transitioned into it. I ate all over the vegan spectrum, including 100 percent whole-food plant-based (WFPB) vegan, no-oil vegan, and even high-carb vegan. My aches subsided, and overall, I felt better when I did not eat animal products.

Then in 2015, I launched VegInspired.com to document the delicious vegan recipes John and I were trying in our kitchen. I was passionate about showing the world how easy and tasty plant-centered meals could be. I found joy sharing our experiments in the kitchen, connecting with others through comments and the VegInspired social channels, and finding like-minded people with whom to share recipes, strategies, and lifestyle tips. Since then, VegInspired has blossomed into a business where I offer lifestyle coaching and write cookbooks like this one!

But in December 2019, after I stepped on the scale and read my highest weight ever, I knew something needed to change. I had been feeling groggy, and my clothes were getting tighter. Of course, while I was aware of the health benefits of eating whole plant-based foods, I had slipped more toward the vegan junk foods. I was a bit embarrassed by my weight gain because I would always share with people how light and healthy I felt eating a plant-based diet. Obviously, eating even vegan junk food isn't that healthy! I was determined to lose the weight and show myself (and others) the power of plants. I transitioned to a high-starch, low-fat, whole-food, plant-based way of eating with goals to lose 35 pounds, feel more alert, and get into better physical shape so I could hike and bike longer trails without feeling out of breath. My journey wasn't perfect, but I worked diligently to create daily habits (positive talk and affirmation, meal planning, eating whole plant-based foods, and light exercise) that aligned with my goals. After six months, I celebrated losing 35 pounds, kicking the grogginess, and being able to go on long, beautiful hikes again!

I have been able to maintain that weight loss through continued focus on my daily habits. I am satisfied with the delicious plant-based meals I eat, I am happy with my results, and I can hike and ride my bike for much longer distances without feeling fatigued. I recognize that the plant-based diet may not be the best approach for everyone—and I encourage you to consult a physician or medical professional before any major dietary changes—but it worked wonders for me. That said, it's important to understand that plant-based eating is a lifestyle, not a short-term diet. I knew what felt best for me and wanted to make this change for my own well-being. Do what makes you feel like the best version of yourself, no matter what the numbers.

After going through this process, I found certain strategies—like accountability, meal planning, easy meal ideas, mindset work, and affirmations—to be critical for success. I created a plant-based lifestyle coaching program (VegInspired.com/coaching) to help others alleviate the stress or anxiety often felt when making lifestyle changes. I lead people through their journey, meeting them where they are and guiding them to where they want to go. That is how I want you to think of this book: a guide to support a lifestyle change. No matter where you are coming from (lifelong carnivore, vegan junk foodie, or experienced plant-based eater), something in this book will help you make healthier eating easier and more enjoyable. This book starts with practical tips in chapter 1, and then each recipe chapter follows a strategy, such as "no-cook meals" or "one-pot meals," to help you easily eat more plants. Some of my favorite time-saving recipes are the Peanut Butter and Jelly Oatmeal Cups (page 28), Tofu Chilaquiles (page 50), Coconut Curry Soup (page 54), Sheet Pan Fajitas (page 109), and Stuffed Sweet Potatoes (page 110).

I hope that you find inspiration and enjoyment with these recipes and that they become your tried-and-true plant-based favorites.

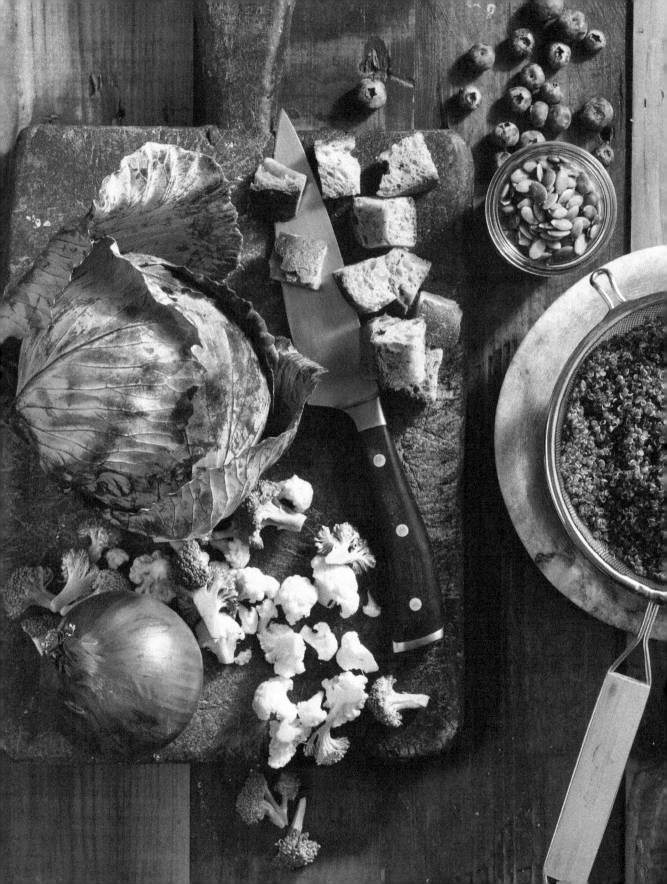

CHAPTER 1

Easy Plant-Based Eating

Welcome to *Super Easy Plant-Based Cookbook*. I am thrilled to share with you my secrets for easy plant-based eating. You may have picked up this book to start eating more plants for health reasons or because you are curious about a plant-based diet. Whatever your reason, you're probably looking for quick, easy, plant-based recipes that you can incorporate into your lifestyle. Whether you are new to plant-based eating or a seasoned herbivore, these quick recipes will help you eat more plants and save time in the kitchen! This chapter will explore the definition of a plant-based diet, tips about eating plant-focused meals, and most important, tricks to save time and energy when cooking plant-based meals.

Health Made Simple

Plant-based eating has gained popularity in recent years as people find the positive impacts outweigh their fears of reducing their consumption of animal products and processed foods. As I mentioned, my story is similar. As I learned how delicious plant-focused meals could be, I had less trouble reducing the animal products I ate because I was excited to try new plant-based meals. It's no secret that eating a diet focused on whole plant ingredients increases your health. Mainstream news outlets and publications are sharing the information presented by plant-based diet advocates like Dr. Michael Greger, of NutritionFacts.org and the author of *How Not to Die and How Not to Diet*, and Dr. Caldwell Esselstyn, author of *Prevent and Reverse Heart Disease*. In fact, Dr. Kim Williams, American College of Cardiology president emeriti, has spoken out many times in the media and in journals to discuss the benefits of plant-focused diets, and has even declared himself vegan for his health.

GO-TO PLANT-BASED MEALS

This book is all about simplicity! Take the complication out of eating plant-based by focusing on the grains or vegetables you already love and simply adding more plants. Some of my favorite, unpretentious meals are a quick bowl of oats or a smoothie made with plant-based milk or yogurt for breakfast, a veggie sandwich or bowl of soup for lunch, and roasted vegetable bowls or pasta with store-bought pasta sauce and frozen vegetables for dinner. I find that when I overcomplicate my meals, I get frustrated and sick of cooking. For a jump start on eating more plants, try these recipes:

- Rainbow Vegetable Sandwiches (page 43)
- Tex-Mex Taco Salad (page 39)
- Apple-Cinnamon Breakfast Quinoa (page 46)
- Vegetable Hummus Pasta (page 83)
- Barbecue Sweet Potato Bowl (page 19)

Plant-based eating is growing in popularity because it works. People suffering from heart disease, diabetes, and some cancers have noticed positive impacts on their health after adopting a plant-based diet, as noted by Dr. Esselstyn in his work with patients at the Cleveland Clinic. Consistently eating nutrient-dense meals low in cholesterol and saturated fat (both of which are found in high quantities in animal products) helps prevent and reduce (and in some cases reverse) symptoms of cardiovascular disease and diabetes.

So why don't more people make the switch? Assumptions that plant-based meals are fancy or expensive, difficult to cook, and flavorless seem to be the top reasons. However, eating more plants doesn't have to be any of those. It can be as simple as adding more greens to your pasta, swapping out chicken broth for vegetable broth, or adding beans or grains to your favorite salad. This chapter will give you my super easy plant-based eating tricks to make delicious, simple, and budget-friendly meals!

About the Plant-Based Diet

A plant-based diet focuses primarily on eating fruits, vegetables, whole grains, and legumes. Some define this as an official diet with restrictions (no animal products or processed foods), while others view it more as a general guide toward eating more plant-based foods (and may still incorporate animal products or processed foods into their diet). Below, I'll explain how this book defines "plant-based."

100 Percent Plants

All the recipes in this book are 100 percent plant based. There will be no animal products in any of them. Additionally, I encourage you to make conscious choices when buying ingredients to avoid those containing animal products (such as dairy in pasta sauce or anchovies in dressings).

Whole Foods

The recipes in this book focus on whole-food ingredients. Focusing on whole foods means using ingredients in their natural states and avoiding overly processed or packaged foods. Some lightly processed foods, such as whole-grain bread and pasta, tofu, and unsweetened plant-based milk, are okay in moderation. Look at "Health and Convenience" (page 6) to better understand what this book considers healthy versus unhealthy processed items.

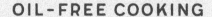

OIL-FREE COOKING

Cooking without oil takes a little practice, but you will find your groove and be a pro in no time. Here are ways to sauté and roast without oil.

Sauté: Bring your pan to medium-high heat, add the vegetables, and reduce the heat to medium. Add a splash of water or vegetable broth to prevent burning. Keeping a close eye on your vegetables and using a nonstick pan (I stand by my cast-iron pan!) will help, but don't be afraid to add water. If you add too much water, your vegetables might steam a little, but you can just drain off the excess water before serving.

Roast: This is my favorite simple cooking method. I use a baking sheet lined with parchment paper or a silicone baking mat and high heat (around 400°F). Just season your prepped vegetables with a little salt and pepper, then place them in the preheated oven. No mess, no fuss, and the vegetables are delicious on their own or with a healthy sauce.

Salt, Oil, and Sugar

Earlier, I mentioned the whole-food, plant-based (WFPB) diet, which takes a plant-based diet one step further by eliminating salt, oils, and refined sugar (SOS). These ingredients have become hugely problematic in the standard American diet (SAD). Many processed foods contain large amounts of salt and sugar, which can lead to a cycle of craving these ingredients and developing health problems. In this book, you will find minimal use of these ingredients.

SALT

Some of my recipes call for a minimal amount of salt during the cooking process. You may substitute Salt-Free Spice Blend (page 14) in the recipes or at the table.

OIL

The recipes in this cookbook will not use oil or products containing oil. My stance is that of the three, oil poses the most significant threat to our health because it is a leading cause of heart disease. Additionally, oil is a highly pro-cessed ingredient, and this book will focus on whole-food ingredients for healthy sources of fat. Review the "Oil-Free Cooking" sidebar (page 4) for more informa-tion on cooking without oil.

SUGAR

The recipes in this cookbook will primarily use natural sweeteners such as fruits (dates, bananas, and unsweetened applesauce) or maple syrup.

Find Your Easy

The stress-free meals in this book are organized by different easy strate-gies, including:

→ **No Cook:** Meals that require no heat to prepare.
→ **30 Minutes:** Meals that can be prepared in 30 minutes or fewer.
→ **5 Ingredient:** Meals that use five ingredients or less, not including water, salt (or my Salt-Free Spice Blend, page 14), or pepper.
→ **One Pot:** Meals that require only one vessel (pot, pan, etc.).

Everyone's definition of easy is different, and what is easy on one day might not be easy on another. The beauty of this cookbook is that you have multi-ple ways to achieve tasty meals. For example, you might find that you stick to 30-minute meals on weekdays and one-pot meals on the weekends, since they may need to cook longer.

While some recipes may fall within a few categories, they are found in the category that makes them most notable. For example, the Vegetable Hummus Pasta (page 83) is a one-pot meal, but what makes it so amazing is that it only requires five ingredients. Therefore, you will find that recipe in chapter 5: 5-Ingredient Meals (page 69).

This book primarily focuses on main meals, but I've included some break-fast recipes and a bonus chapter on treats and snacks. Additionally, the index, organized by meal type, allows you to look for specific types of recipes, like "breakfast" or "salad," for even greater ease. Finally, you'll find labels to help those with dietary restrictions—gluten-free, nut-free, and soy-free. Just be sure to check the labels on products (like gluten-free for oats) to make sure they truly fit your dietary needs.

HEALTH AND CONVENIENCE

When eating more plant-focused meals, you will use fewer highly processed ingredients. In this book, you won't see packaged snacks; processed vegan meat and cheese alternatives; or dairy-free butter, ice cream, etc. You will find minimally processed, healthy options that will provide flavor and texture to your meals. Whole-grain bread, cereal, and pasta; tofu and tempeh; unsweetened plant-based milk; low-ingredient sauces (e.g., oil-free marinara); and some condiments (e.g., organic ketchup, seasoned rice vinegar, mustard,) will play a role in these recipes.

In chapter 2: Homemade Staples (page 13), you will find recipes you can make ahead of time and keep on hand for speedy meals. Any recipe that uses a homemade staple will also have a store-bought alternative to keep your cooking effortless.

Additionally, while tofu and tempeh are great meat alternatives, don't count out beans! Beans are high in fiber and protein and work well to add a hearty texture to dishes like tacos (Black Bean and Sweet Potato Tacos, page 59) and curries (Mango-Ginger Chickpea Curry, page 106).

Finally, there are some lightly processed brands of convenience foods that are worth mentioning. Engine 2 products (found exclusively online), Sunshine Burger, and many nut-based dairy alternatives or spreads (like Notcho Nocheez and Kite Hill) are slightly processed. However, they may contain less (or no) oil, salt, or sugar, making them a healthy alternative in moderation.

Below are some additional healthier substitutes worth mentioning.

PROCESSED ITEM	HEALTHIER ALTERNATIVE
Meat alternatives	Homemade burgers, tofu, and tempeh
Dairy-free cheeses	Nutritional yeast, oil-free cheese spreads
Vegan butter	Vegetable broth, avocado, or hummus
Vegan ice cream	Cherry Nice Cream (page 134)

Smart Shopping

Smart shopping is the key to success. By purchasing ingredients that lend themselves to quick and easy cooking, you set yourself up for a win. Below are my top smart shopping ingredients to purchase, so you are ready to cook anytime.

Canned Beans: Dried beans are cheap and nutritious but take time to cook for use in a recipe. Having various canned beans in your pantry will help on those nights you don't have time to boil dried beans. Look for BPA-free canned goods, low-sodium or no-salt-added varieties, and buy organic when possible.

Dried Herbs and Spices: Keeping your spice rack full of your favorite spices helps flavor your food in a pinch. Onion and garlic powders can be used in place of fresh to save time prepping and sautéing. Dried herbs are more potent then fresh, so use a simple conversion: roughly 1 teaspoon of dried herbs for every 1 tablespoon of fresh herbs.

Frozen Vegetables: Nothing says "quick prep" quite like a bag of frozen vegetables. All the peeling, chopping, and dicing is done for you, meaning you simply need to open the bag. Frozen starches, like potatoes and squash, can reduce cooking time since they are partially cooked before they are frozen. Vegetables such as frozen broccoli or cauliflower make it incredibly easy to add nutrients to your stir-fries and other dishes, and if chopping onions makes you cry, look for frozen diced onions.

Minced Ginger and Garlic: These store-bought prepped ingredients make adding fresh aromatics, essential for adding flavor, a breeze. And cleanup is a snap since there is no garlic press or zester to wash.

Quick-Cooking Starches: Parboiled grains or rice speed up your cooking time and usually don't contain added salt or preservatives. If you opt for precooked grains, be sure to check the ingredients for added salt and preservatives.

Plant-Based Pro Tips

The recipes in this cookbook have you covered in terms of ease and deliciousness. Here I wanted to include some of my pro tips and strategies to help you make eating more plants an integrated part of your lifestyle.

YOUR SECRET PANTRY ARSENAL

Your pantry arsenal is a collection of frequently used ingredients available to help you make healthy and quick meals in no time. Besides my old standby ingredients—rice, canned beans, frozen vegetables, and tofu—I keep a specific group of ingredients in my pantry that enhance my meals' flavors. Here are some of my favorites:

Bragg liquid aminos: This salty and savory condiment is perfect when you want to add some flavor without directly adding table salt. It is wonderful spritzed on air-popped popcorn with a sprinkle of nutritional yeast.

Lemon and lime juice: These are must-haves. Just a splash of juice can brighten your tacos or freshen up a salad. I prefer it bottled for longer shelf life; just check that there are no added ingredients.

Lite coconut milk: From soups to desserts to curries, coconut milk is a must-have for adding creaminess. Make straightforward curry by mixing coconut milk with a store-bought curry paste.

Nutritional yeast: This deactivated yeast is often used in plant-based cooking to add a buttery or cheesy flavor.

Tahini: This paste made from sesame seeds is an excellent base for creamy sauces. It's also my secret ingredient in baked goods because it adds a decadent flavor and airy texture.

Vegetable broth: This is essential as a base for soups and sauces when time is limited. It can enhance flavors and give your meals that "cooked all day" taste. I like to use a low-sodium vegetable broth.

Vinegar: This is great for jazzing up a salad or bringing balance to a recipe. I keep a couple of my favorites—balsamic, rice, and apple cider—in my pantry to use throughout my recipes. A simple salad dressing can be made by combining seasoned rice vinegar and a drizzle of tahini.

Meal Plan

Meal planning is my number one tip for becoming a pro with plant-based eating. When you plan your meals, you save not only save time but also money. Simply write down and schedule the recipes you intend to cook. Visit VegInspired.com/menuplan to download my weekly meal planning template.

Prep Ahead

I like to look at prepping ahead in a few different ways. You can prep entire meals, or you can prep ingredients, such as grains or potatoes, to build different meals throughout the week. Look for the "Easy Prep" label throughout the book to find recipes that require five minutes or less of prep time.

Bowls on the Fly

By far, my favorite meals are bowls. They come together so fast and are full of flavor. Build your bowl by adding prepped vegetables, beans or chickpeas, and a quick drizzle of tahini or vinegar to a base of greens or grains. So simple!

Store-Bought Fallbacks

We all know that delivery comes in handy when time is tight, but those meals aren't typically very healthy. To combat the urge for delivery, I like to keep whole-wheat pita bread in the freezer and a jar of oil-free pizza sauce in the pantry. I'll top it with whatever veggies I have on hand, and will have a quick mess-free pizza in minutes.

Upcycled Leftovers

What treasures do you have in your refrigerator right now? Last night's chili can become today's loaded sweet potato, or roasted veggies can become a delicious taco filling. Try using different sauces or dressings from chapter 2 (page 13) to change your meals' flavors, and suddenly your food is going twice as far! See my Upcycled Leftovers chart (page 10) for some more ideas.

Gadget Guru

The recipes in this cookbook don't rely on kitchen gadgets, but they are worth mentioning as they relate to time-saving tips. Tools like a rice cooker and salad spinner help you prep satisfying ingredients in no time, so you can eat healthy on even the busiest night.

Upcycled Leftovers

RECIPE	UPCYCLE IDEA 1	UPCYCLE IDEA 2
Lemony Kale Salad (page 31)	Pair this with roasted vegetables, potatoes, and/or beans for a tangy taco topping.	Pair this with a simple veggie burger for a unique twist on the standard burger.
Mediterranean-Inspired Picnic Salad (page 36)	Add the leftovers of this salad to cooked pasta or cooked farro for an amped up leftover meal.	Pair this with mixed greens and wrap in a whole-grain tortilla or pita for a fun sandwich.
Cauliflower Scramble (page 49)	Pair the savory-sweet cauliflower with a baked sweet potato or russet potato for a loaded potato.	Pair this with crispy fresh cabbage and oil-free corn tortillas for a unique twist on a taco.
Turmeric Tempeh Stir-Fry (page 62)	Pair this with roasted potatoes, fresh cabbage, and avocado with whole-grain tortillas or pita for a fun wrap or sandwich.	Pair with scrambled tofu for a protein-packed breakfast scramble. Eat alongside whole-grain toast.
Barbecue Beans on Toast (page 71)	These beans can be paired with rice or potatoes for a unique bowl. I like to add red onions, cilantro, and a drizzle of mustard to create a barbecue bowl.	Place the beans in a whole-grain bun or wrap for a simple barbecue sandwich; add sliced pickles and onions to complement the meal.
Four-Can Chili (page 101)	Pair this with baked sweet potatoes or russet potatoes for a fun loaded potato. You can add all your favorite chili toppings.	Chili dogs! Pair this with a carrot dog (VegInspired. com/carrot-dogs) and your favorite chili dog toppings.

RECIPE	UPCYCLE IDEA 1	UPCYCLE IDEA 2
Sheet Pan Scrambled Tofu and Potatoes (page 96)	Pair the tofu and potatoes with oil-free tempeh bacon (VegInspired.com/plant-based-tempeh-bacon) and whole-grain toast or a tortilla for an easy breakfast sandwich or wrap. Add salsa and guacamole for a taco-inspired breakfast sandwich or wrap.	Pair this with salsa or tomatoes and spices to create a variation of the Tofu Chilaquiles (page 50) or One-Pot Shakshuka (page 100).
Sheet Pan Fajitas (page 109)	Pair the roasted veggies with refried beans, Lemony Kale Salad (page 31), and a drizzle of tahini in a whole-grain or oil-free corn tortilla for a flavorful taco or wrap.	Pair this with Aromatic Yellow Rice (page 22) for a fajita bowl.
Stuffed Sweet Potatoes (page 110)	Mash the leftover sweet potatoes and black beans with chopped leftover veggies and fill a whole-grain tortilla for a flavorful quesadilla. Cook in a nonstick skillet for 3 to 5 minutes per side until golden brown.	Pair with baby spinach (or your favorite green) for a roasted bean and veggie salad.

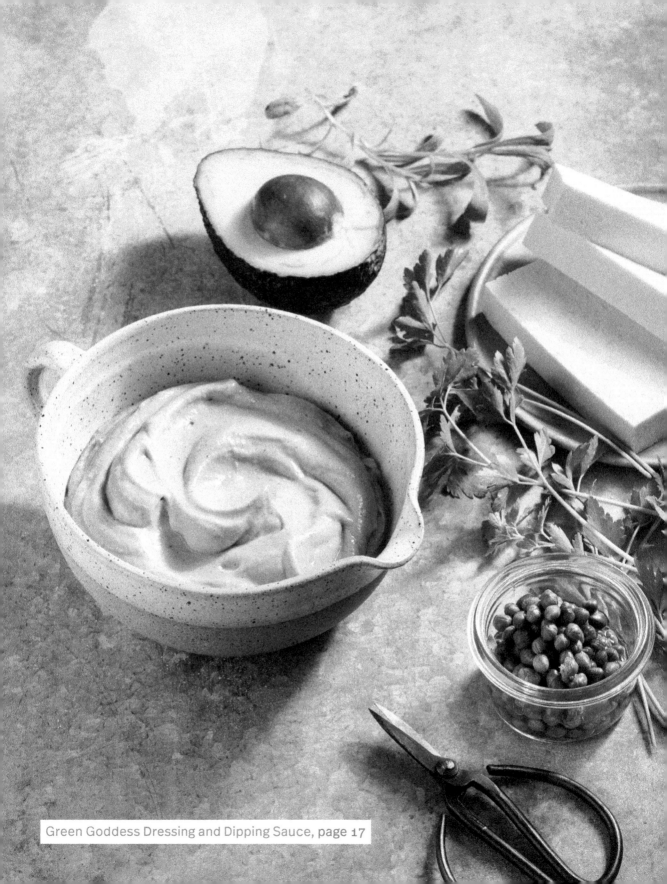

Green Goddess Dressing and Dipping Sauce, page 17

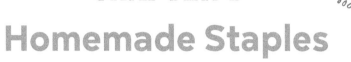

CHAPTER 2

Homemade Staples

Salt-Free Spice Blend

30 MINUTES | EASY PREP | GLUTEN-FREE | NO COOK | NUT-FREE | ONE POT | SOY-FREE

MAKES ABOUT 4 TABLESPOONS PREP TIME: 5 minutes

This is my go-to spice blend whenever I want to add a pop of flavor to a dish without added salt. I repurposed a spice jar to keep a batch of this on hand to sprinkle on my popcorn, plain rice, and Savory Avocado Toast (page 70). It works in just about every recipe in place of salt.

1 tablespoon nutritional yeast

1 tablespoon onion powder

1 teaspoon ground coriander

1 teaspoon ground cumin

1 teaspoon dried parsley

½ teaspoon dried thyme

½ teaspoon freshly ground black pepper

½ teaspoon garlic powder

½ teaspoon dried dill

¼ teaspoon turmeric

¼ teaspoon smoked paprika

In a small bowl, thoroughly mix the nutritional yeast, onion powder, coriander, cumin, parsley, thyme, pepper, garlic powder, dill, turmeric, and paprika. Store in an airtight container.

PER SERVING (¼ TEASPOON): Calories: 1; Total fat: 0g; Total carbs: 0g; Fiber: 0g; Sugar: 0g; Protein: 0g; Sodium: 0mg

Maple-Mustard Dressing

5 INGREDIENT · 30 MINUTES · EASY PREP · GLUTEN-FREE · NO COOK · NUT-FREE
ONE POT · SOY-FREE

MAKES ABOUT ½ CUP **PREP TIME:** 5 minutes

This dressing is a sweet, tangy, and perfectly thick and creamy accent for your vegetables. I enjoy this on a hearty kale salad or drizzled on my roasted vegetables. The seasoned rice vinegar imparts a tangy and slightly sweet flavor that sends this mustard dressing over the top. It is the star of the show in my Broccoli, Chickpea, and Walnut Salad (page 33).

4 tablespoons spicy brown mustard

4 tablespoons pure maple syrup

2 teaspoons seasoned rice vinegar

2 teaspoons tahini

In a small bowl, whisk together the mustard, maple syrup, vinegar, and tahini. Store in an airtight container in the refrigerator.

INGREDIENT TIP: Dijon mustard will also work well in this recipe if you cannot find a suitable spicy brown mustard.

PER SERVING (2 TABLESPOONS): Calories: 77; Total fat: 2g; Total carbs: 15g; Fiber: 1g; Sugar: 12g; Protein: 1g; Sodium: 177mg

Go-To Bowl Sauce

5 INGREDIENT **30 MINUTES** **EASY PREP** **GLUTEN-FREE** **NO COOK** **NUT-FREE**
ONE POT

MAKES ABOUT 1 CUP   PREP TIME: 5 minutes

Bowls are my jam! I love to toss together various ingredients to create a quick and filling meal. But what really jazzes me up is a flavorful saucy component. I think a good sauce can turn last night's leftovers into tonight's showstopper. This simple (and blender-free) tahini sauce is just the ticket with its savory and sweet tang.

½ cup tahini

1 teaspoon miso paste

½ cup water

2 tablespoons seasoned
   rice vinegar

¼ teaspoon onion powder

¼ teaspoon
   ground ginger

1. In a small bowl, whisk together the tahini and miso paste until the miso paste dissolves.

2. Add the water, vinegar, onion powder, and ground ginger and whisk until it's combined, creamy, and smooth. Store in an airtight container in the refrigerator.

INGREDIENT TIP: Tahini thickens as you add water, so continue to whisk until a creamy and smooth texture appears. Tahini can vary in thickness; you may need to reduce (or increase) the amount of water to achieve your desired consistency.

PER SERVING (2 TABLESPOONS): Calories: 92; Total fat: 8g; Total carbs: 4g; Fiber: 2g; Sugar: 0g; Protein: 3g; Sodium: 44mg

Green Goddess Dressing and Dipping Sauce

`30 MINUTES` **EASY PREP** `GLUTEN-FREE` `NO COOK` **NUT-FREE** **ONE POT**

MAKES ABOUT 1½ CUPS PREP TIME: 5 minutes

Pull out your blender for this easy, creamy dressing. Standard green goddess dressing calls for mayonnaise and sour cream, neither of which are part of a plant-based diet. I use tofu and avocado to create the perfect velvety texture, then add simple ingredients to round out the flavors and pump up the dressing's traditional green hue. I love this as a dip for fresh vegetables, a dressing for salads, or a sauce on one of my bowls.

½ block firm tofu

6 tablespoons freshly squeezed lemon juice

1 avocado, pitted and peeled

2 tablespoons unsweetened soy milk

1 tablespoon Dijon mustard

1 tablespoon tarragon

1 tablespoon dried parsley

1 tablespoon capers, drained

1 tablespoon liquid aminos

1 scallion, green and white parts, coarsely chopped

¼ teaspoon freshly ground black pepper

⅛ teaspoon garlic powder

1. In a blender, combine the tofu, lemon juice, avocado, soy milk, mustard, tarragon, parsley, capers, liquid aminos, scallion, pepper, and garlic powder.

2. Blend for about 30 seconds until smooth and creamy. Store in an airtight container in the refrigerator.

INGREDIENT TIP: No liquid aminos? Replace with low-sodium gluten-free soy sauce or tamari.

PER SERVING (2 TABLESPOONS): Calories: 42; Total fat: 3g; Total carbs: 3g; Fiber: 1g; Sugar: 0g; Protein: 2g; Sodium: 35mg

Weeknight Tomato Sauce

MAKES ABOUT 4 CUPS PREP TIME: 5 minutes **COOK TIME:** 15 minutes

This rich, flavorful tomato sauce works well anywhere you need it—on pizza, pasta, rice, and more. It is one of those recipes that is so easy, you'll wish you'd learned about it sooner. Store-bought sauces can be a challenge; I often find myself reading labels of pasta sauces and getting frustrated that they contain oil, tons of sodium, or loads of sugar. Using fresh basil in this recipe brightens up the tomatoes without the sugar, and no oil is necessary. A pinch of salt helps enhance the tomato flavor, but it can easily be omitted.

1 (28-ounce) can crushed tomatoes

1 cup loosely packed fresh basil

2 tablespoons nutritional yeast

2 teaspoons onion powder

1 teaspoon garlic powder

¼ teaspoon salt

1. In a medium saucepan over medium heat, combine the tomatoes, basil, nutritional yeast, onion powder, garlic powder, and salt.

2. Bring the sauce to a simmer and cook for about 15 minutes, until fragrant. Store in an airtight container in the refrigerator.

VARIATION TIP: This weeknight tomato sauce works well on pasta, whole grains like farro, or your favorite plant-based pizza dough. I like to use it on Vegetable Pita Pizzas (page 58).

PER SERVING (½ CUP): Calories: 36; Total fat: 0g; Total carbs: 8g; Fiber: 2g; Sugar: 4g; Protein: 2g; Sodium: 258mg

Barbecue Sauce

30 MINUTES **EASY PREP** **GLUTEN-FREE** **NUT-FREE** **ONE POT** **SOY-FREE**

MAKES ABOUT 2½ CUPS **PREP TIME:** 5 minutes **COOK TIME:** 15 minutes

Making homemade barbecue sauce is a game changer. Many store-bought sauces are laden with sugars, salt, or oil, and reading labels can be so time-consuming. This recipe is ready in about 20 minutes and can be used for dressing grilled vegetables or topping a veggie burger. It's also used in the Barbecue Sweet Potato Bowl (page 111).

1 cup water

1 cup tomato paste

¼ cup pure maple syrup

3 tablespoons apple cider vinegar

2 tablespoons molasses

1 tablespoon smoked paprika

1 teaspoon garlic powder

1 teaspoon onion powder

½ teaspoon freshly ground black pepper

1. In a medium saucepan, bring the water to a rolling boil over high heat. Reduce the heat to low, then whisk in the tomato paste, maple syrup, vinegar, molasses, paprika, garlic powder, onion powder, and pepper. Cover and simmer for 10 minutes.

2. Remove from the heat and cool for about 30 minutes before transferring to an airtight container. Store in the refrigerator for up to 1 week.

INGREDIENT TIP: I prefer to use blackstrap molasses because it adds a nutrient punch of magnesium and iron to my meals. Often it is noted on the label if the molasses is blackstrap or not.

PER SERVING (2 TABLESPOONS): Calories: 29; Total fat: 0g; Total carbs: 7g; Fiber: 1g; Sugar: 5g; Protein: 1g; Sodium: 9mg

Quick Pickled Vegetables

GLUTEN-FREE NO COOK NUT-FREE SOY-FREE

PREP TIME: 10 minutes, plus 1 hour to pickle **SERVES:** 4

I love pickles, but many on the market use Yellow 5 for coloring. I try to avoid artificial colors, so I came up with these quick pickled veggies that work just as well. They're perfect for sandwiches, salads, bowls, and snacking.

For the cucumbers

2 cups sliced cucumbers
  (¼-inch-thick rounds)
½ cup seasoned
  rice vinegar
½ cup boiling water
½ teaspoon freshly
  ground black pepper
Pinch red pepper flakes
  (optional)

For the carrots

1 cup (1-inch-long)
  carrot sticks
¼ cup boiling water
¼ cup seasoned
  rice vinegar
¼ teaspoon dried dill

1. **Make the cucumbers:** Place the cucumbers in a shallow bowl with a lid.

2. In a separate small bowl, whisk together the vinegar, boiling water, black pepper, and red pepper flakes (if using). Carefully pour the mixture over the cucumbers, ensuring all of the vegetables are submerged.

3. **Make the carrots:** Place the carrots in a shallow bowl with a lid.

4. In a separate small bowl, whisk together the boiling water, vinegar, and dill. Carefully pour the mixture over the carrots, ensuring all of the vegetables are submerged.

5. Place lids over the bowls and refrigerate the pickled vegetables for at least 1 hour (or up to 24 hours for best flavor). Store for up to 5 days.

INGREDIENT TIP: Cutting your vegetables in uniform shape and size will help with consistency in flavor and texture. You can try different shapes (rounds or sliced lengthwise) for various applications. Quartering baby carrots is much easier than prepping whole ones!

PER SERVING: Calories: 30; Total fat: 0g; Total carbs: 5g; Fiber: 2g; Sugar: 3g; Protein: 0g; Sodium: 24mg

Roasted Potatoes

GLUTEN-FREE NUT-FREE ONE POT SOY-FREE

PREP TIME: 10 minutes **COOK TIME:** 50 minutes **SERVES:** 4

Buttery roasted potatoes were one of my favorite side dishes. While plant-based butter exists on the market, they are typically vegetable oil-based, which does not align with my preference for oil-free meals or with a minimally processed plant-based diet. In this oil-free version, the combination of vegetable broth and nutritional yeast yields a delightful buttery flavor without the oil. The addition of smashed garlic adds a nice flavor, too, though I don't recommend eating the garlic unless you are trying to ward off vampires.

2 pounds yellow potatoes, cut into 1-inch pieces

½ cup vegetable broth

1 tablespoon nutritional yeast

1 teaspoon Salt-Free Spice Blend (page 14)

1 teaspoon dried rosemary

¼ teaspoon freshly ground black pepper

2 garlic cloves, smashed

1. Preheat the oven to 400° F.

2. In a roasting pan or large glass baking dish, combine the potatoes and broth. Add the nutritional yeast, spice blend, rosemary, pepper, and garlic, stirring to combine.

3. Roast for 40 to 50 minutes, stirring at least once halfway through, until the potatoes are browned and tender. Enjoy warm.

INGREDIENT TIP: This recipe works very well with halved baby potatoes. Their consistent shape presents well, and they cook evenly.

SHORTCUT: In a pinch, use a store-bought salt-free spice blend in place of the homemade blend.

PER SERVING: Calories: 177; Total fat: 0g; Total carbs: 40g; Fiber: 5g; Sugar: 2g; Protein: 5g; Sodium: 14mg

Aromatic Yellow Rice

5 INGREDIENT **EASY PREP** **GLUTEN-FREE** **NUT-FREE** **ONE POT** **SOY-FREE**

PREP TIME: 5 minutes **COOK TIME:** 45 minutes **SERVES:** 4

I tossed a bay leaf in with my rice in the rice cooker one day and was wowed by the added flavor. I decided to play around with other spices and herbs and created this flavorful and brightly colored rice. Turmeric is a super spice thanks to curcumin's nutritional power, which is said to reduce everything from aches and pains to inflammation and cardiovascular ailments. I'd say that is super, too!

2 cups water

1 cup brown rice

½ teaspoon turmeric

½ teaspoon
   onion powder

1 bay leaf

¼ teaspoon garlic powder

¼ teaspoon freshly
   ground black pepper

1. In a medium saucepan, bring the water to a boil over high heat.

2. Reduce the heat to low. Add the rice, turmeric, onion powder, bay leaf, garlic powder, and pepper. Cover and simmer for 45 minutes, or until the rice is no longer chewy.

3. Remove and discard the bay leaf and serve.

INGREDIENT TIP: I typically follow the package instructions for cooking rice and simply add the spices when I add my rice. You can also add these ingredients to your rice cooker; these quantities work for up to 3 cups of rice.

PER SERVING: Calories: 175; Total fat: 2g; Total carbs: 37g; Fiber: 2g; Sugar: 0g; Protein: 4g; Sodium: 3mg

Savory Braised Tempeh

5 INGREDIENT **EASY PREP** **FREEZES WELL** **GLUTEN-FREE** **NUT-FREE**

PREP TIME: 5 minutes **COOK TIME:** 30 minutes **SERVES:** 2 to 4

Tempeh, the lesser-known soy product, is made by fermenting soybeans, which binds them into a block or cake form. It is more nutritionally dense than tofu as it uses the whole bean, making it popular in whole-food, plant-based recipes. Recipes that use tempeh often call for it to be boiled or steamed to help neutralize the flavor, which is why this recipe works perfectly to reduce the bitterness and impart a savory flavor. You also may wonder if the poultry seasoning is plant-based, and the answer is yes! Most are a simple spice blend of herbs, such as sage, rosemary, and black pepper, that give your tempeh a familiar flavor.

1 (8-ounce) package tempeh, cut into ½-inch-thick slices

1 cup vegetable broth

1½ tablespoons poultry seasoning

1 teaspoon liquid aminos

1. Place the tempeh into a medium skillet so that none of the slices overlap.

2. In a small bowl, mix together the broth, poultry seasoning, and liquid aminos. Pour the broth mixture over the tempeh, making sure each piece is submerged.

3. Over medium-high heat, bring the mixture to a boil. Reduce the heat to medium-low and gently simmer for about 20 to 30 minutes, or until the liquid is absorbed. Halfway through, use a spoon to baste or redistribute the liquid over tempeh slices that may have poked out as the liquid absorbs and evaporates.

4. Store the tempeh in an airtight container in the refrigerator for up to 5 days.

VARIATION TIP: A soy-free alternative is canned young jackfruit that has been drained, shredded, and rinsed well.

PER SERVING: Calories: 118; Total fat: 7g; Total carbs: 7g; Fiber: 0g; Sugar: 0g; Protein: 11g; Sodium: 184mg

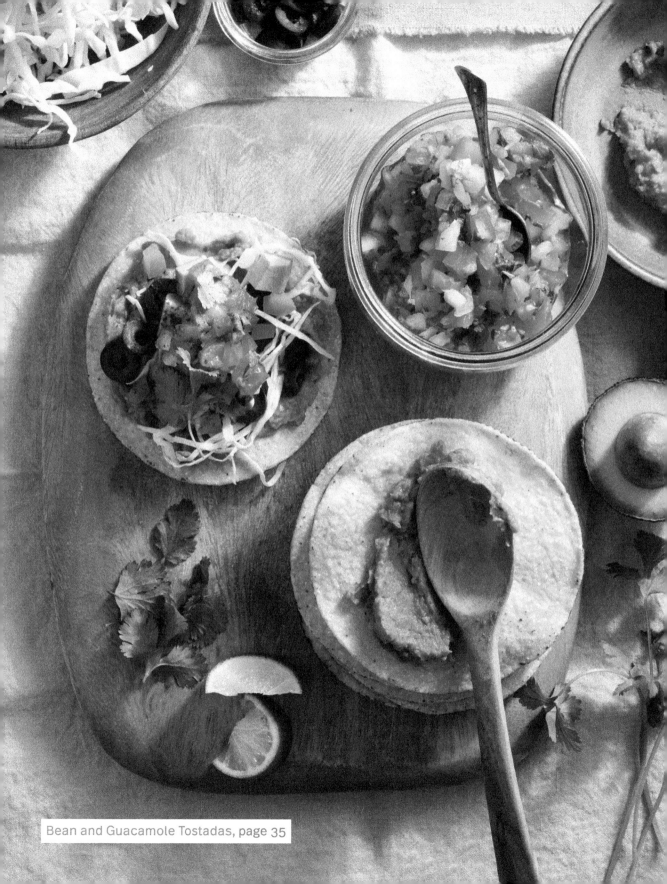

Bean and Guacamole Tostadas, page 35

CHAPTER 3
No-Cook Meals

Banana-Raspberry Smoothie Bowl

30 MINUTES   GLUTEN-FREE   NO COOK   ONE POT   SOY-FREE

PREP TIME: 10 minutes **SERVES:** 4

Is there anything better than a meal that tastes like dessert? This healthy yet decadent smoothie bowl is a mouthwatering delight any time of the day. Creamy, sweet bananas paired with the tart raspberries make this bowl delicious and beautiful. The smoothie is scrumptious on its own, but I love to add oats and some crunchy nuts or seeds to jazz it up a bit. Or try a drizzle of date syrup!

6 cups frozen banana chunks

1 cup frozen raspberries

2 tablespoons nut butter of choice

1 heaping tablespoon ground flaxseed

½ teaspoon almond extract

½ cup unsweetened plant-based milk

1. In a food processor, pulse the banana chunks until they have a crumbly texture.

2. Add the raspberries, nut butter, flaxseed, and almond extract and process to combine.

3. While the food processor is running, slowly add the milk. As the liquid mixes in, the frozen mixture should begin to form a ball. Scrape the sides of the food processor and continue to blend until no chunks remain and the mixture has a thick smoothie or soft-serve ice cream texture. Serve.

INGREDIENT TIP: To prepare frozen bananas, peel ripe bananas and cut them into 1-inch chunks. Lay the bananas on a parchment-lined plate or baking sheet that fits in your freezer. Freeze for 4 to 6 hours, transfer to an airtight container, and store in the freezer until ready to use.

PER SERVING: Calories: 297.5; Total fat: 7g; Total carbs: 60g; Fiber: 10g; Sugar: 30g; Protein: 6g; Sodium: 19mg

The Fruit Smoothie Formula

5-INGREDIENT 30 MINUTES GLUTEN-FREE NO COOK NUT-FREE ONE POT
SOY-FREE

PREP TIME: 10 minutes **SERVES:** 2

I love a good smoothie, and for a long time, I drank one every day for breakfast on my commute to work. I would mix up whatever fruit and plant-based milk I had in my kitchen and see which combinations I preferred. Banana-blueberry and mango-strawberry were my favorites. Bananas always seem to be a go-to for smoothies, but frozen mangos can add a delightful creaminess when bananas aren't available.

2 cups unsweetened
   plant-based milk
2 cups chopped fresh or
   frozen fruit
2 tablespoons ground
   flaxseed
1 cup ice (optional)

In a blender, combine the milk, fruit, flaxseed, and ice (if using) and purée for 30 seconds to 1 minute, until smooth and creamy. Serve.

INGREDIENT TIP: You can make this gluten-, nut-, or soy-free depending on the plant-based milk you use. If you want it to be free of all three, use pea milk or a seed-based milk like hemp.

PER SERVING: Calories: 189; Total fat: 7g; Total carbs: 24g; Fiber: 6g; Sugar: 13g; Protein: 9g; Sodium: 124mg

Peanut Butter and Jelly Oatmeal Cups

5 INGREDIENT GLUTEN-FREE NO COOK SOY-FREE

MAKES 6 CUPS PREP TIME: 5 minutes, plus 2 hours to chill

What a classic duo, peanut butter and jelly. I love the idea of break-fast cookies, but they often need to be baked; I like recipes I can make quickly and have ready to go for a quick breakfast the next day. In this recipe, a base of nut butter and oats works flawlessly to create little cups to hold fruity jam.

1 cup rolled oats

½ cup smooth natural
  peanut butter

2 tablespoons pure maple
  syrup

2 tablespoons ground
  flaxseed

Pinch salt

6 tablespoons low-sugar
  or sugar-free jelly or jam

1. Line a muffin tin with six liners. In a large bowl, combine the oats, peanut butter, maple syrup, flaxseed, and salt.

2. Add 3 tablespoons of the oat mixture to each liner in the prepared muffin tin.

3. Using a 1-tablespoon scoop, firmly press the oat mixture into each liner, leaving a well in the middle.

4. Cover and refrigerate for at least 2 hours.

5. Add 1 tablespoon of your favorite jelly or jam to each cup and enjoy!

PREPARATION TIP: These little cups are so much fun for breakfast. I recommend making them in batches and transferring them to an airtight container; the liners will keep them from sticking together.

PER SERVING: Calories: 260; Total fat: 13g; Total carbs: 27g; Fiber: 4g; Sugar: 13g; Protein: 7g; Sodium: 101mg

Muesli and Yogurt Breakfast Parfait

`30 MINUTES` `EASY PREP` `GLUTEN-FREE` `NO COOK` `SOY-FREE`

PREP TIME: 5 minutes **SERVES:** 2

Muesli is basically loaded oats. The neat part about it is that you can use whatever nuts, seeds, and dried fruit you like, so feel free to get creative. Sometimes I use goji berries in place of raisins (or in addition to raisins). I've also added hemp hearts or sunflower seeds to some of my muesli mixes. Mix and match to discover your own favorite combos!

1 cup rolled oats

2 tablespoons unsweet-
  ened raisins

2 tablespoons sliced
  almonds

2 tablespoons chopped
  walnuts

2 tablespoons cacao nibs

2 tablespoons ground
  flaxseed

1 teaspoon date sugar

1 cup plant-based yogurt

1 cup berries

1. In a medium bowl, mix together the oats, raisins, almonds, walnuts, cacao nibs, flaxseed, and sugar.

2. In two small serving bowls, layer ½ cup of muesli mix, ½ cup of yogurt, and ½ cup berries. Serve.

PREPARATION TIP: Double or triple your batch of muesli to keep on hand for quick meals or snacks. Muesli can be eaten with plant-based milk like cereal.

SHORTCUT: You can also use a store-bought muesli in a pinch.

PER SERVING: Calories: 420; Total fat: 16g; Total carbs: 57g; Fiber: 10g; Sugar: 14g; Protein: 13g; Sodium: 18mg

Paradise Island Overnight Oatmeal

GLUTEN-FREE NO COOK NUT-FREE ONE POT SOY-FREE

PREP TIME: 10 minutes, plus 4 hours to chill **SERVES:** 2

Overnight oats are like a present you give to yourself. Waking up to a grab-and-go breakfast (or having one in the refrigerator for an effort-less snack) is exactly what you need on a busy day. The bright and ambrosial flavors in this recipe are sure to make you smile on a cold wintry day. Oatmeal is a hearty and satiating meal that keeps you full and provides the heart-healthy, fiber-filled benefits of plant foods!

2 cups rolled oats

2 cups unsweetened plant-based milk

½ cup diced fresh or frozen mango

½ cup fresh or frozen pineapple chunks

1 banana, sliced

1 tablespoon pure maple syrup

1 tablespoon chia seeds

1. In a large bowl, mix together the oats, milk, mango, pineapple, banana, maple syrup, and chia seeds.

2. Cover and refrigerate overnight, or for at least 4 hours. Serve.

PREPARATION TIP: Make this recipe early in the week—or even make a double recipe—and separate it into covered, single-serving containers so you'll have 2 to 4 breakfasts ready to eat.

PER SERVING: Calories: 638; Total fat: 13g; Total carbs: 109g; Fiber: 16g; Sugar: 31g; Protein: 21g; Sodium: 123mg

Lemony Kale Salad

5 INGREDIENT 30 MINUTES GLUTEN-FREE NO COOK NUT-FREE ONE POT
SOY-FREE

PREP TIME: 10 minutes **SERVES:** 4

Zesty lemon paired with bold garlic gives this robust green salad a pop of flavor. Massaging the kale helps break down its sturdy structure, yielding a softer, more appealing texture. Kale is loaded with antioxidants and is an excellent source of vitamin C and vitamin K. This recipe is sure to have you adding more kale to your weekly meals.

2 tablespoons freshly
  squeezed lemon juice
½ tablespoon pure maple
  syrup
1 teaspoon minced garlic
5 cups chopped kale

In a large bowl, whisk together the lemon juice, maple syrup, and garlic. Add the kale, massage it in the dressing for 1 to 2 minutes, and serve.

PREPARATION TIP: Make sure to thoroughly massage the kale with the dressing ingredients. This will give the kale a beautiful texture and properly incorporate the lemon and garlic flavors.

PER SERVING: Calories: 19; Total fat: 0g; Total carbs: 4g; Fiber: 1g; Sugar: 2g; Protein: 1g; Sodium: 8mg

Green Goddess Chopped Salad

PREP TIME: 15 minutes **SERVES:** 4

I used to love a chopped salad coated in a thick and creamy dressing when I dined out in my pre-vegan days. Now, I typically opt for vinegar or lemon slices on the side of my restaurant salads to steer clear of commercial dressings full of oil and other undesirable ingredients. But at home, I can control my ingredients and make myself a quick and easy chopped with a dreamy creamy dressing. Many of the ingredients in this salad can be purchased prepped right from your grocer's produce aisle, so this meal-worthy salad can be ready in minutes!

2 cups loosely packed chopped lettuce

1 cup baby greens, chopped

1 cup chopped broccoli florets

1 cup rinsed cooked chickpeas

½ cup shredded cabbage

½ cup chopped cucumbers

¼ cup chopped carrots

¼ cup chopped red bell pepper

¼ cup sliced radish

¼ cup chopped walnuts or sliced almonds

¼ to ½ cup Green Goddess Dressing and Dipping Sauce (page 17)

1. In a large bowl, using tongs, mix together the lettuce, greens, broccoli, chickpeas, cabbage, cucumbers, carrots, bell pepper, radish, and walnuts.

2. Add the dressing and toss to coat evenly, then serve.

SHORTCUT: In a pinch, use a store-bought plant-based dressing in place of Green Goddess Dressing and Dipping Sauce.

PER SERVING: Calories: 292; Total fat: 15g; Total carbs: 32g; Fiber: 11g; Sugar: 8g; Protein: 13g; Sodium: 239mg

Broccoli, Chickpea, and Walnut Salad with Maple-Mustard Dressing

30 MINUTES **GLUTEN-FREE** **NO COOK** **ONE POT** **SOY-FREE**

PREP TIME: 10 minutes **SERVES:** 4

Broccoli and mustard are a powerhouse pair in both taste and nutritional benefits. Mustard is high in an enzyme called myrosinase, which maximizes the absorption of a compound in broccoli called sulforaphane. Too much science? In a nutshell: Eat your broccoli, cooked and uncooked, with a bit of mustard, and you can amp up the anticancer and antidiabetic properties of the broccoli!

2 cups chopped broccoli florets

1 (15-ounce) can chickpeas, drained and rinsed

½ cup chopped walnuts

1 teaspoon dried dill

¼ teaspoon onion powder

1 batch Maple-Mustard Dressing (page 15)

1. In a large bowl, using a rubber spatula or wooden spoon, mix together the broccoli, chickpeas, and walnuts.

2. Sprinkle on the dill and onion powder.

3. Add the dressing and toss the broccoli mixture to evenly coat, then serve immediately.

SHORTCUT: Use a store-bought vegan honey-mustard dressing (such as Follow Your Heart brand) or your favorite whole-food, plant-based oil-free dressing (such as Cindy's Kitchen brand).

PER SERVING: Calories: 269; Total fat: 13g; Total carbs: 34g; Fiber: 12g; Sugar: 15g; Protein: 9g; Sodium: 313mg

Artichoke and Avocado Rolls

30 MINUTES NO COOK NUT-FREE ONE POT SOY-FREE

PREP TIME: 10 minutes **SERVES:** 4

This recipe is loosely inspired by lobster rolls. I wanted to create a decadent plant-based sandwich that had the luxury associated with the richness of lobster. I used artichokes for the "lobster" texture and avocado for its delicious, buttery creaminess. The recipe calls for dulse flakes (seaweed), which are often found in the Asian foods section near the nori sheets or kelp granules. Both crumbled nori sheets and kelp granules can be used in place of dulse; simply halve the amount.

2 avocados, pitted and peeled

1 (14-ounce) can quartered arti-chokes, drained

3 tablespoons thinly sliced scallions, green and white parts

2 tablespoons freshly squeezed lemon juice

1 tablespoon diced celery

1 tablespoon nutritional yeast

½ teaspoon dulse flakes

¼ teaspoon freshly ground black pepper

⅛ teaspoon salt

⅛ teaspoon garlic powder

4 whole-grain burger or hot dog buns

1. In a small bowl, mash the avocados to a creamy paste.

2. Stir in the artichokes, scallions, lemon juice, celery, nutritional yeast, dulse flakes, pepper, salt, and garlic powder.

3. Place a ½ cup portion of the mixture on each of the four buns, then serve.

INGREDIENT TIP: When selecting avocados, pick ones that have a slight give near the stem. Store them in the refrigerator until soft enough to use. If you can't find slightly soft ones, you can buy firm ones and just let them soften on the counter.

PER SERVING: Calories: 310; Total fat: 18g; Total carbs: 35g; Fiber: 12g; Sugar: 4g; Protein: 9g; Sodium: 324mg

Bean and Guacamole Tostadas

`30 MINUTES` `GLUTEN-FREE` `NO COOK` `NUT-FREE` `SOY-FREE`

PREP TIME: 10 minutes **SERVES:** 4

These tostadas are like a pizza, flat taco, and nachos all mixed into one. The day I found baked tostada shells in the grocery store was game-changing. I was looking for a vessel for guacamole that didn't have oil and was thrilled to learn that tostadas are baked without oil (only a bit of salt) and are available at most grocers. They perfectly satisfied my chips and guacamole craving and quickly became a staple in my pantry.

1 (15.5-ounce) can fat-free refried beans

1 teaspoon chili powder

3 tablespoons freshly squeezed lime juice, divided

8 baked tostadas

¾ cup shredded cabbage

½ cup sliced black olives

½ cup diced fresh tomatoes

1 avocado, pitted, peeled, and diced

½ cup salsa

½ cup chopped fresh cilantro

1. In a small bowl, mix together the refried beans, chili powder, and 1 tablespoon of lime juice.

2. Spread about 2 tablespoons of the refried bean mixture evenly over each tostada.

3. Divide the cabbage, olives, tomatoes, and avocado evenly between the tostadas. Then top each with an even amount of the salsa and the remaining 2 tablespoons of lime juice.

4. Garnish with the cilantro, then serve.

INGREDIENT TIP: My favorite refried beans are the 365 Everyday Value brand roasted chili and lime refried pinto beans from Whole Foods, which have no oil. Refried beans are traditionally made with lard or oil, so double-check the ingredients when purchasing.

PER SERVING: Calories: 324; Total fat: 15g; Total carbs: 41g; Fiber: 12g; Sugar: 4g; Protein: 10g; Sodium: 924mg

Mediterranean-Inspired Picnic Salad

`30 MINUTES` `GLUTEN-FREE` `NO COOK` `NUT-FREE`

PREP TIME: 20 minutes **SERVES:** 4

Nothing excites me more than a loaded vegetable salad tossed with a tasty and tangy dressing. This salad recipe came about when I wanted a fast and satiating picnic salad but didn't want to boil pasta or pearled farro. I mixed all the other pasta salad ingredients with a tangy dressing and voilà! A meal ready in minutes. You could easily add 1 to 2 cups of cooked whole-grain pasta or 1 cup of cooked farro to increase the fiber in this salad; if you choose to do this, just remember to double your dressing to accommodate the added ingredients.

For the salad

2 cups loosely packed chopped lettuce

1 (15-ounce) can chickpeas, drained and rinsed (reserve liquid for dressing)

1 (15-ounce) can quartered artichokes, drained

1 cup chopped cucumbers

½ cup chopped fresh tomatoes

¼ cup thinly sliced red onion, rinsed

¼ cup kalamata olives, sliced (optional)

¼ cup oil-free roasted red pepper, sliced (optional)

1. **Make the salad:** In a large bowl, mix together the lettuce, chickpeas, artichokes, cucumbers, tomatoes, onion, olives (if using), and red pepper (if using).

2. **Make the dressing:** In a measuring cup, whisk together the aquafaba and miso paste until the miso paste is dissolved. Add the vinegar, tahini, lemon juice, nutritional yeast, oregano, garlic powder (if using), and red pepper flakes (if using).

For the dressing

⅓ cup aquafaba (reserved chickpea liquid)

½ tablespoon miso paste

2 tablespoons red wine vinegar

1 tablespoon tahini

½ tablespoon freshly squeezed lemon juice

½ tablespoon nutritional yeast

¼ teaspoon dried oregano

⅛ teaspoon garlic powder (optional)

⅛ teaspoon red pepper flakes (optional)

3. Add the dressing to the salad, ½ cup at a time, and stir the ingredients together with a rubber spatula or wooden spoon until well coated.

4. Store the salad in an airtight container in the refrigerator until ready to serve.

INGREDIENT TIP: Aquafaba is the juice from a can of chickpeas. I often will drain the chickpeas, reserving the liquid to use in dressings. The aquafaba provides a thicker and more neutral replacement for oil than vegetable broth or water.

SHORTCUT: You can cut down on prep time by purchasing precut veggies.

PER SERVING: Calories: 171; Total fat: 5g; Total carbs: 27g; Fiber: 10g; Sugar: 5g; Protein: 9g; Sodium: 289mg

Buffalo Tofu Salad

PREP TIME: 5 minutes **SERVES:** 4

Buffalo-flavored anything is top on my list of favorites. I use Frank's RedHot, but there are lower sodium hot sauce options on the market if you prefer. This salad is tantalizing when layered between two whole-grain bread slices, wrapped in a whole-grain tortilla or pita, or used as a spread for crackers. I love that it blends buffalo sauce's spiciness and the creaminess of a dressing into one palate-pleasing salad.

1 (14-ounce) block firm tofu

½ cup shredded carrots

¼ cup finely chopped celery

2 tablespoons chopped celery leaves

2 tablespoons sliced scallions, green and white parts

½ cup hot sauce

¼ cup apple cider vinegar

2 tablespoons tahini

¼ teaspoon garlic powder

¼ teaspoon dried dill

⅛ teaspoon salt

Whole-grain bread, for serving

1. In a medium bowl, mash the tofu with a fork. Add the carrots, celery, celery leaves, and scallions and stir to combine.

2. Stir in the hot sauce, vinegar, tahini, garlic powder, dill, and salt, then serve with bread.

INGREDIENT TIP: I like to keep Food For Life Ezekiel bread products on hand for sandwiches. Their products use whole grains to create a nutrient-dense and less processed bread option, which aligns with the plant-based diet. They are often found in the grocery store's freezer section, so they will keep in your freezer and be an excellent staple for a go-to sandwich (and you only need to take out the bread you want to use it). When I am ready to use my Ezekiel bread, I carefully separate the slices with a knife and lightly toast them.

PER SERVING: Calories: 203; Total fat: 13g; Total carbs: 9g; Fiber: 4g; Sugar: 2g; Protein: 17g; Sodium: 297mg

Tex-Mex Taco Salad

PREP TIME: 10 minutes **SERVES:** 4

Tacos are my absolute favorite meal, but they can also be time-consuming to make and prep, so I created this loaded taco salad with all of the flavors but none of the cooking. I love that I can find many of these ingredients already sliced and ready to use, which cuts down on my prep.

½ cup raw cashews

¼ cup water

6 tablespoons salsa, divided

1 (15-ounce) can black beans, drained and rinsed

2 cups shredded lettuce

1 cup frozen corn, thawed

1 cup diced fresh tomatoes

½ cup sliced black olives

1 large avocado, pitted, peeled, and diced

1 low-sodium taco seasoning packet

1 tablespoon freshly squeezed lime juice

1. In a high-efficiency blender, combine the cashews, water, and 4 tablespoons of salsa and blend to a creamy, smooth texture.

2. In a large bowl, mix together the beans, lettuce, corn, tomatoes, olives, avocado, the remaining 2 tablespoons of salsa, the taco seasoning, lime juice, and cashew cream until thoroughly combined. Serve immediately.

PREPARATION TIP: If you do not have a high-efficiency blender, soak the cashews in warm water for 1 hour before blending in your less powerful blender to prevent the motor from burning out. Discard the water before use.

PER SERVING: Calories: 357; Total fat: 19g; Total carbs: 40g; Fiber: 12g; Sugar: 6g; Protein: 13g; Sodium: 380mg

Spring Rolls with Pistachio Sauce

30 MINUTES **GLUTEN-FREE** **NO COOK** **SOY-FREE**

PREP TIME: 15 minutes **SERVES:** 4

These sweet and spicy vegetable spring rolls are a reliable tasty meal for me. I love the varied textures in this recipe and that I can make them ahead of time for lunch on the go. When I make them in advance, I place a lettuce leaf between the rolls so that the rice papers don't stick together.

1 large cucumber

1 large carrot

4 ounces fresh basil

½ cup shelled unsalted pistachios

1 serrano or jalapeño pepper, halved and seeded

3 tablespoons rice vinegar

8 rice paper wrappers

1. Halve the cucumber crosswise, then cut each half into 16 (¼-inch-wide) sticks.

2. Quarter the carrot lengthwise, then cut each quarter into 4 (¼-inch-wide) sticks.

3. In a food processor, combine the basil, pistachios, serrano, and vinegar and purée, adding 1 tablespoon of water at a time as needed to create a thick sauce.

4. Pour warm water into a shallow bowl. Dip one rice paper wrapper into the water until moistened, about 5 seconds (do not let it soak). Place the wrapper on a work surface and let sit for about 30 seconds, until pliable. Dollop about 2 tablespoons of the pistachio sauce on the wrapper and add two cucumber sticks and two carrot sticks. Lift one side of the wrapper and fold it over the filling, then tuck it under the filling. Fold in the sides and roll up the spring roll. Repeat with the remaining ingredients.

5. Plate the rolls and drizzle more sauce on top. Store the sauce in an airtight container in the refrigerator for up to 5 days.

INGREDIENT TIP: This pistachio sauce is versatile! Use the sauce as a vegetable dip, dollop it over a bowl of beans, greens, and grains, or spread it over whole-grain toast.

PER SERVING: Calories: 209; Total fat: 7g; Total carbs: 30g; Fiber: 4g; Sugar: 4g; Protein: 6g; Sodium: 105mg

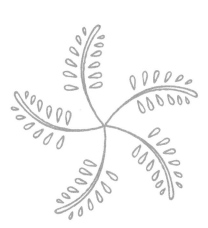

Avocado Black Bean Medley

PREP TIME: 10 minutes **SERVES:** 4

This fiber-packed bean and kale salad is brightened up with creamy avocados, juicy cherry tomatoes, and lime juice. I love the simplicity of using canned beans to create a nutrient-dense punch to my salads. Black beans are probably my favorite because of their versatility and their high antioxidant count, but you can use any bean you like.

2 cups tightly packed finely chopped kale

Juice of 1 lime

1 teaspoon minced garlic

½ teaspoon red pepper flakes

½ teaspoon salt

¼ teaspoon ground cumin

1 (15-ounce) can black beans, drained and rinsed (or 1½ cups cooked black beans)

2 avocados, pitted, peeled, and diced

2 cups quartered cherry tomatoes

¼ cup finely chopped red onion

1. Place the kale in a large bowl.

2. In a small bowl or measuring cup, whisk together the lime juice, garlic, red pepper flakes, salt, and cumin. Pour the dressing over the kale. Toss to coat or use your hands to massage the dressing into the kale to soften it.

3. Add the beans, avocados, tomatoes, and onion. Toss gently, then serve.

VARIATION TIP: Use low-sodium pinto beans or corn to replace the black beans.

PER SERVING: Calories: 270; Total fat: 15g; Total carbs: 30g; Fiber: 14g; Sugar: 4g; Protein: 9g; Sodium: 306mg

Rainbow Vegetable Sandwiches

30 MINUTES **EASY PREP** **GLUTEN-FREE** **NO COOK** **NUT-FREE** **SOY-FREE**

PREP TIME: 5 minutes **SERVES:** 2

As a kid, my favorite sandwich was sliced cucumbers and mayonnaise. I think my favorite part of the sandwich was the fact that my mom would get so excited to make them for me. I remember her telling me how they were her favorite sandwiches . . . and what little girl doesn't want to be just like her mom? This sandwich is a grown-up version; I use creamy mashed avocados as an alternative to mayo, and I added a few more vegetables for some additional texture and flavor.

½ cup shredded cabbage

2 tablespoons seasoned rice vinegar

Freshly ground black pepper

4 whole-grain bread slices

1 avocado, pitted, peeled, and quartered

Salt

½ cup sliced cucumbers

½ cup sliced cooked beets

¼ cup shredded carrots

4 onion slices

4 tomato slices

1. In a small bowl, combine the cabbage, vinegar, and a pinch pepper.

2. Place the bread on a plate, then place a quarter of the avocado on each piece. Mash the avocado, then season with salt and pepper.

3. Layer the cucumbers, beets, dressed cabbage, carrots, onion, and tomato on two of the bread slices. Top each with the remaining two bread slices, then serve.

INGREDIENT TIP: Use canned or precooked beets found in your grocer's produce section for a quick version of this sandwich. Double-check the ingredients for a low-salt option when available.

PER SERVING: Calories: 373; Total fat: 17g; Total carbs: 47g; Fiber: 13g; Sugar: 10g; Protein: 12g; Sodium: 350mg

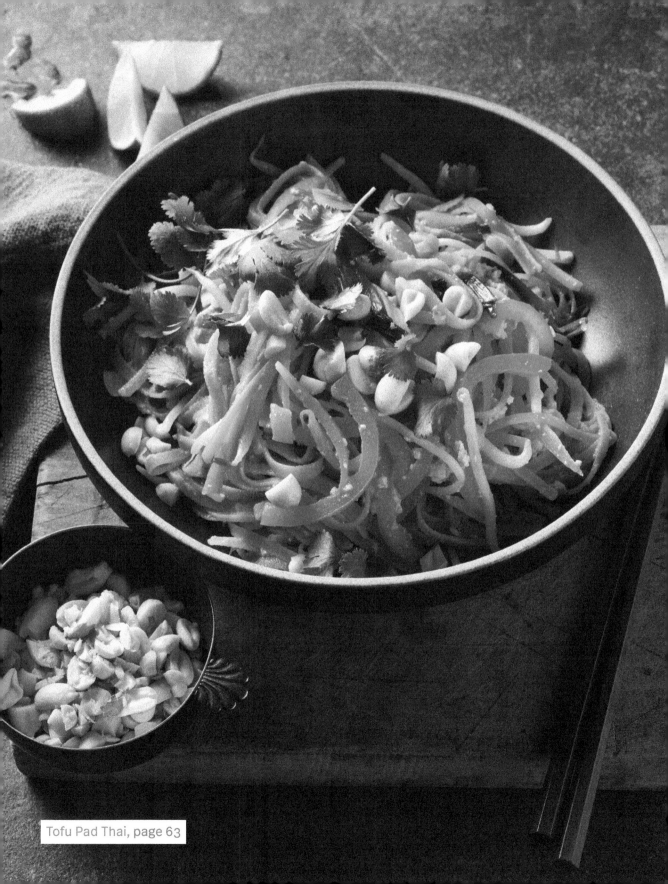

Tofu Pad Thai, page 63

CHAPTER 4
30-Minute Meals

Apple-Cinnamon Breakfast Quinoa

30 MINUTES   EASY PREP   GLUTEN-FREE   SOY-FREE   ONE POT

PREP TIME: 5 minutes   **COOK TIME:** 20 minutes   **SERVES:** 4

This quinoa tastes just like apple pie. I created this dish one chilly fall morning, and my entire house smelled of the holidays. Enjoying the scents wafting through my home is a major reason I make this for breakfast! Such a treat to wake up to. Using quinoa in this dish adds a punch of protein that gives you a heart-healthy breakfast.

- 1 large apple, diced (about 2 cups)
- 8 large dates, pitted and chopped (½ cup)
- 1 teaspoon vanilla extract
- ½ teaspoon ground cinnamon
- 2 cups water
- 1 cup quinoa
- 4 tablespoons pure maple syrup
- ¼ cup chopped pecans

1. In a medium saucepan over medium heat, combine the apple, dates, vanilla, and cinnamon and sauté for about 5 minutes, until apple is starting to soften and the mixture is fragrant. Add 1 to 2 tablespoons of water as needed to prevent burning.

2. Add the water and quinoa to the pan. Bring to a rolling boil, then reduce the heat to low. Cover and simmer for 15 minutes, until the quinoa is cooked and liquid is absorbed.

3. Remove the pan from the heat and let stand for 5 minutes. Serve with 1 tablespoon of maple syrup and 1 tablespoon of chopped nuts.

VARIATION TIP: Don't love apples? Try pears instead.

PER SERVING: Calories: 340; Total fat: 8g; Total carbs: 63g; Fiber: 7g; Sugar: 30g; Protein: 7g; Sodium: 6mg

Carrot Cake Oatmeal

30 MINUTES **GLUTEN-FREE** **SOY-FREE**

PREP TIME: 10 minutes   **COOK TIME:** 15 minutes   **SERVES:** 2

I would describe this oatmeal as cozy and nostalgic. I love the warm cinnamon, spicy ginger, and fragrant nutmeg—the combination reminds me of cake! Oats have been a staple on my plant-based journey because of their high fiber and satiating nature. Adding the pecans further aids the satiation with that punch of protein. Eating a bowl of oats in the morning for breakfast always keeps me full and happy until lunch.

¼ cup pecans

1 cup finely shredded carrot

½ cup rolled oats

1¼ cups unsweetened plant-based milk

1 tablespoon pure maple syrup

1 teaspoon ground cinnamon

1 teaspoon ground ginger

¼ teaspoon ground nutmeg

2 tablespoons chia seeds

1. In a small skillet over medium-high heat, toast the pecans for 3 to 4 minutes, stirring, until browned and fragrant (watch closely, as they can burn quickly). Pour the pecans onto a cutting board and roughly chop them. Set aside.

2. In an 8-quart pot over medium-high heat, combine the carrot, oats, milk, maple syrup, cinnamon, ginger, and nutmeg. Bring to a boil, then reduce the heat to medium-low. Cook, uncovered, for 10 minutes, stirring occasionally.

3. Stir in the chopped pecans and chia seeds. Serve immediately.

PREPARATION TIP: This oatmeal can also be prepared by mixing all the ingredients in a sealable container and refrigerating it overnight. The texture will be chewier and denser, but overnight oats are an easy way to meal prep for a no-brainer breakfast.

PER SERVING: Calories: 388; Total fat: 19g; Total carbs: 45g; Fiber: 12g; Sugar: 13g; Protein: 13g; Sodium: 117mg

Plant-Powered Pancakes

30 MINUTES EASY PREP FREEZES WELL NUT-FREE SOY-FREE

PREP TIME: 5 minutes **COOK TIME:** 15 minutes **SERVES:** 4

Who doesn't love a stack of pancakes in the morning? These easy pancakes, made with simple ingredients, are excellent served with a drizzle of maple syrup or mixed fruit. Keeping with the plant-based focus, this recipe uses applesauce to retain moisture and keep the pancakes light and fluffy.

1 cup whole-wheat flour

½ teaspoon ground cinnamon

1 teaspoon baking powder

1 cup unsweetened plant-based milk

½ cup unsweetened applesauce

¼ cup pure maple syrup

1 teaspoon vanilla extract

1. In a large bowl, combine the flour, cinnamon, and baking powder.

2. Stir in the milk, applesauce, maple syrup, and vanilla until no dry flour is left and the batter is smooth.

3. Heat a large nonstick skillet or griddle over medium heat. For each pancake, pour ¼ cup of batter onto the hot skillet. Cook for 1 to 2 minutes, until bubbles form on top and the sides begin to brown. Flip and cook for 1 to 2 minutes, until browned.

4. Repeat until all of the batter is used, then serve.

VARIATION TIP: To add a fruity twist to this recipe, place a few blueberries on the batter right after pouring it into the pan.

PER SERVING: Calories: 204; Total fat: 2g; Total carbs: 42g; Fiber: 5g; Sugar: 16g; Protein: 6g; Sodium: 35mg

Cauliflower Scramble

30 MINUTES GLUTEN-FREE SOY-FREE

PREP TIME: 15 minutes **COOK TIME:** 15 minutes **SERVES:** 4

Look no further for a savory breakfast. The warm spices and rich coconut aminos bring the umami in this vegetable-packed breakfast. Coconut aminos can be substituted for soy sauce in many recipes; they provide a similar flavor, are gluten-free, and have 65 percent less sodium. The flavor is subtle with a hint of sweetness; they definitely don't taste like coconut!

1 onion, diced

3 garlic cloves, minced

1 green bell pepper, coarsely chopped

1 red bell pepper, coarsely chopped

1 large head cauliflower, cored and chopped into ½-inch florets

1 teaspoon ground turmeric

¼ cup nutritional yeast

¼ teaspoon ground nutmeg

¼ teaspoon cayenne pepper

¼ teaspoon freshly ground black pepper

1 tablespoon coconut aminos

1 (15-ounce) can chickpeas, drained and rinsed

1. In a large nonstick skillet over medium heat, combine the onion, garlic, and green and red bell peppers. Cook for 2 to 3 minutes, stirring, until the onion is translucent but not browned. Add 1 to 2 tablespoons of water as needed to prevent burning.

2. Add the cauliflower and toss to combine. Cover the skillet and cook for 5 to 6 minutes, or until the cauliflower is fork-tender.

3. While the cauliflower is cooking, in a small bowl, stir together the turmeric, nutritional yeast, nutmeg, cayenne, and black pepper. Set aside.

4. Evenly sprinkle the coconut aminos over the cauliflower mixture and stir to combine. Stir in the spice mixture. Stir in the chickpeas and cook, uncovered, for 5 minutes to warm. Serve.

PREPARATION TIP: Sautéing without oil is one of the tricks you'll use often throughout this book. Adding water to the pan, 1 tablespoon at a time, helps keep onions and garlic from sticking or burning, but still allows them to sauté.

PER SERVING: Calories: 166; Total fat: 2g; Total carbs: 31g; Fiber: 10g; Sugar: 10g; Protein: 9g; Sodium: 243mg

Tofu Chilaquiles

30 MINUTES **EASY PREP** **GLUTEN-FREE** **NUT-FREE** **ONE POT**

PREP TIME: 5 minutes **COOK TIME:** 10 minutes **SERVES:** 2 to 4

Traditional chilaquiles start by frying tortillas in oil and then simmering them in a red sauce such as salsa. Frying is not aligned with a plant-based way of eating, so in this recipe we start with baked tostadas. For a soy-free option, substitute a can of drained and rinsed chickpeas or pinto beans for the tofu.

1 (14-ounce) firm tofu, drained and crumbled

1 tablespoon onion powder

½ teaspoon ground cumin

¼ teaspoon salt

¼ teaspoon garlic powder

¼ teaspoon turmeric

1 (15-ounce) can black beans, drained and rinsed

1 (16-ounce) jar salsa

4 baked tostadas, roughly broken

2 tablespoons chopped fresh cilantro, plus more for garnish

¼ cup sliced onion, rinsed

2 to 4 lime wedges

1 avocado, pitted, peeled, and chopped

1. In a large nonstick sauté pan or skillet over medium heat, combine the tofu, onion powder, cumin, salt, garlic powder, and turmeric. Cook, stirring frequently, for 3 to 5 minutes, until heated through. Add 1 to 2 tablespoons of water as needed to prevent burning.

2. Add the beans, salsa, and tostadas, carefully submerging the tostadas in the liquid. Reduce the heat to medium-low. Simmer for about 5 minutes, until the tostadas soften. Remove from the heat and stir in the cilantro.

3. Serve warm with the onion, lime, and avocado. Garnish with cilantro.

VARIATION TIP: You can make this spicy by using a hot salsa.

PER SERVING: Calories: 343; Total fat: 15g; Total carbs: 41g; Fiber: 13g; Sugar: 6g; Protein: 18g; Sodium: 1,048mg

Vegan "Toona" Salad

30 MINUTES GLUTEN-FREE NUT-FREE NO COOK ONE POT SOY-FREE

PREP TIME: 10 minutes **SERVES:** 4

This vegan salad filling is ready in minutes, no appliances needed! A trusty potato masher or a fork will do the trick. Mashing the chickpeas creates a wonderful texture for the salad while the onion and celery bring in a balanced crunch. If you have it on hand, a pinch of dulse or kelp granules will give this salad a subtle from-the-sea taste.

2 (15-ounce) cans chickpeas, drained and rinsed

1 avocado, pitted and peeled

½ cup chopped red onion

¼ cup chopped celery

2 tablespoons Dijon mustard

1 ½ tablespoons freshly squeezed lemon juice

½ tablespoon pure maple syrup

1 teaspoon garlic powder

1. In a large bowl, combine the chickpeas and the avocado. Using a fork or a potato masher, smash them down until the majority of the chickpeas have been broken apart. (You don't want to purée the chickpeas; just smash them enough so they're able to absorb the rest of the flavors of the dish.)

2. Stir in the onion, celery, mustard, lemon juice, maple syrup, and garlic powder, making sure everything is thoroughly combined, and serve.

VARIATION TIP: Vegan "Toona" Salad is great on top of freshly toasted whole-grain bread as a traditional or open-faced sandwich. You may also enjoy adding a juicy slice of tomato, a lettuce leaf, a drizzle of balsamic glaze, or all three.

PER SERVING: Calories: 276; Total fat: 10g; Total carbs: 40g; Fiber: 11g; Sugar: 8g; Protein: 12g; Sodium: 338mg

Lentil Potato Soup

30 MINUTES **EASY PREP** **GLUTEN-FREE** **NUT-FREE** **ONE POT** **SOY-FREE**

PREP TIME: 5 minutes **COOK TIME:** 20 minutes **SERVES:** 4

Potato soup screams comfort food, and this brothy version with lentils and smoked paprika is like a warm hug any time of the year. Lentils' nutritional offerings include high fiber, antioxidants, and protein. They are also a great source of B vitamins, iron, magnesium, potassium, and zinc. They're a budget-friendly and neutral plant-based ingredient!

4 cups vegetable broth

3 cups diced potatoes

1 cup dried brown
   lentils, rinsed

1 tablespoon
   onion powder

1 tablespoon nutritional
   yeast

½ teaspoon smoked
   paprika

¼ teaspoon garlic powder

¼ teaspoon salt

¼ teaspoon freshly
   ground black pepper

⅛ teaspoon celery seed

⅛ teaspoon red
   pepper flakes

1 bay leaf

1. In a large saucepan or Dutch oven over high heat, combine the broth, potatoes, lentils, onion powder, nutritional yeast, smoked paprika, garlic powder, salt, pepper, celery seed, red pepper flakes, and bay leaf. Bring to a boil.

2. Reduce the heat to medium-low. Cover and simmer for 18 to 20 minutes, until the potatoes are knife-tender. Remove and discard the bay leaf. Serve warm.

PER SERVING: Calories: 164; Total fat: 0g; Total carbs: 35g; Fiber: 7g; Sugar: 4g; Protein: 7g; Sodium: 715mg

Cheezy Broccoli Soup

30 MINUTES GLUTEN-FREE

PREP TIME: 10 minutes **COOK TIME:** 15 minutes **SERVES:** 4 to 6

In plant-based cooking, many people miss the cheese they used to eat. In this cozy soup, I use the flavor and texture of cooked squash, the creaminess of blended raw cashews, and the buttery, cheesy flavor of nutritional yeast to create a savory and flavorful soup brimming with vegetables.

1 (9-ounce) bag frozen squash

4 cups vegetable broth, divided

¼ cup nutritional yeast

1 tablespoon onion powder

¼ teaspoon smoked paprika

¼ teaspoon garlic powder

¼ teaspoon freshly ground black pepper

¼ cup raw cashews

1 (10.5-ounce) bag frozen broccoli

1 teaspoon red miso paste

1. In a large saucepan or Dutch oven over high heat, combine the squash, 2 cups of broth, the nutritional yeast, onion powder, smoked paprika, garlic powder, and pepper. Bring to a boil, then cook for 3 to 5 minutes, until the squash is tender.

2. Transfer the solids and at least 1 cup of broth to a high-speed blender. Add the cashews and blend until smooth and creamy.

3. Transfer the blended soup mixture back to the pan. Add the 2 remaining cups of broth and return to a boil. Add the broccoli and miso paste, and simmer for 7 to 10 minutes, until the broccoli is crisp-tender. Serve warm.

PREPARATION TIP: If you have 9 ounces of leftover cooked squash, you can skip step 1 and start by blending the squash with the vegetable broth and spices.

PER SERVING (2 CUPS): Calories: 120; Total fat: 5g; Total carbs: 18g; Fiber: 4g; Sugar: 4g; Protein: 5g; Sodium: 69mg

Coconut Curry Soup

30 MINUTES **EASY PREP** **GLUTEN-FREE** **SOY-FREE**

PREP TIME: 5 minutes **COOK TIME:** 15 minutes **SERVES:** 4

This curry soup hits the spot when you want something warming and a little spicy. The coconut milk and aromatic tandoori seasoning gives it a balanced, gratifying taste. Tandoori seasoning is often used to cook traditional Indian chicken, which is often finished with plain yogurt. To keep this recipe plant-based, we use blended chickpeas to create a thick texture for a soup that eats like a meal.

1 ½ cups vegetable broth

1 (15-ounce) can chickpeas, drained and rinsed

1 (13.5-ounce) can lite coconut milk

1 large carrot, coarsely chopped

1 small red onion, quartered

½ teaspoon tandoori seasoning

½ teaspoon curry powder

¼ teaspoon salt

⅛ to ¼ teaspoon white pepper

1. In a blender or food processor, combine the broth, chickpeas, coconut milk, carrot, onion, tandoori seasoning, curry powder, and salt and blend until smooth.

2. Transfer the soup mixture to a large saucepan or Dutch oven. Bring to a vigorous simmer over medium-high heat (constant small bubbles will form), then reduce the heat to low. Gently simmer for 10 minutes, until the flavors meld. Stir in the pepper just before serving.

PREPARATION TIP: Make your own tandoori seasoning! Combine equal parts paprika, ground coriander, and cayenne pepper.

SHORTCUT: If you have a high-speed blender (such as a Vitamix or Blendtec) you can "cook" this soup in it. Add all of the ingredients and blend at the highest speed for 6 minutes. *Voilà!* Hot soup!

PER SERVING: Calories: 292; Total fat: 21g; Total carbs: 19g; Fiber: 5g; Sugar: 4g; Protein: 6g; Sodium: 292mg

Hot and Sour Tofu Soup

30 MINUTES   EASY PREP   GLUTEN-FREE

PREP TIME: 5 minutes   **COOK TIME:** 15 minutes   **SERVES:** 2

Packed with immune-boosting garlic and ginger, this umami-rich soup is sure to delight your palate. I love that I can make a robust, flavorsome soup in less than 30 minutes. Look for a red chili paste without oil. I have found roasted chile pastes often contain oil.

¼ cup gluten-free tamari or low-sodium soy sauce

2 teaspoons red or yellow miso paste

2 teaspoons red chili paste

1 teaspoon minced garlic

2 teaspoons minced fresh ginger

1 cup sliced mushrooms

3 cups water

1 (12-ounce) package silken tofu

¼ cup crushed unsalted peanuts (optional)

¼ cup chopped scallions, green parts only

1. In a large saucepan over medium-high heat, cook the tamari until it just begins to bubble. Add the miso and mash it with a fork to create a thick slurry. Add the chili paste, garlic, and ginger and cook, stirring frequently, for 3 minutes.

2. Add the mushrooms and water and bring to a boil, then reduce the heat to medium-low. Add the tofu, crumbling it with your fingers and dropping it into the pan. Cover and simmer for 10 minutes.

3. Divide the peanuts (if using) and scallions between two large bowls. Ladle half the soup into each bowl and serve.

VARIATION TIP: Add 1 cup of your favorite frozen veggies (corn, peas, and green beans are nice options) when you crumble in the tofu.

PER SERVING: Calories: 149; Total fat: 7g; Total carbs: 10g; Fiber: 2g; Sugar: 3g; Protein: 16g; Sodium: 1,145mg

Vegetable and Avocado Quesadillas

30 MINUTES **EASY PREP** **NUT-FREE** **ONE POT**

PREP TIME: 5 minutes **COOK TIME:** 10 minutes **SERVES:** 2

The creative filling options for these quesadillas are endless. I've tried adding other vegetables, such as corn, carrots, asparagus, and cabbage, with delicious results. The secret is to cut the vegetables small enough so that the avocado can hold the tortilla together. Another way to kick things up a notch is to substitute pickled jalapeño peppers or sauerkraut for the briny olives.

4 oil-free whole-grain tortillas

2 avocados, pitted, peeled, and mashed

½ cup shredded baby spinach

½ cup broccoli slaw

½ cup thinly sliced red bell pepper

2 tablespoons thinly sliced scallion, green and white parts

2 tablespoons sliced olives

½ cup salsa

½ cup Green Goddess Dressing and Dipping Sauce (page 17)

1. On each tortilla, evenly spread half of the mashed avocado.

2. Divide the spinach, broccoli slaw, bell pepper, scallion, and olives between the tortillas and fold them in half.

3. Heat a large nonstick skillet over medium heat. Gently place the tortillas in the pan and cook for 3 to 5 minutes per side, until tortillas are lightly browned and crisped.

4. Serve with salsa and green goddess dressing.

SHORTCUT: Use a plant-based, store-bought creamy dip in place of green goddess dressing.

PER SERVING: Calories: 394; Total fat: 25g; Total carbs: 37g; Fiber: 14g; Sugar: 4g; Protein: 11g; Sodium: 554mg

Beet Reuben Sandwiches

30 MINUTES NUT-FREE NO COOK

PREP TIME: 10 minutes **SERVES:** 4

Earthy, sweet beets help achieve a delicious flavor profile for this sandwich that is inspired by a traditional Reuben. Beets are an often-forgotten root vegetable, but their health benefits make them a star of the veggie world. They are low in calories and high in fiber, which is beneficial for heart and digestion. Additionally, they are loaded with antioxidants, which are helpful in reducing inflammation.

For the Reuben sauce

¼ block firm tofu, drained

3 tablespoons ketchup

1½ tablespoons apple
   cider vinegar

2 teaspoon Dijon mustard

1 teaspoon water, plus
   more as needed

⅛ teaspoon garlic powder

¼ cup diced pickles

For the sandwiches

8 whole-grain bread
   slices, lightly toasted

2 cups cooked beets,
   warmed and sliced

1 cup sauerkraut

1 teaspoon Salt-Free
   Spice Blend (page 14)

1. **Make the Reuben sauce:** Combine the tofu, ketchup, vinegar, mustard, water, and garlic powder in a blender. Blend until smooth, adding water 1 teaspoon at a time if the texture is too thick. Transfer the sauce to a small bowl and stir in the diced pickles. You should have about 1 cup of sauce.

2. **Make the sandwiches:** On one piece of bread, layer ½ cup of beets, ¼ cup of sauerkraut, ¼ teaspoon of salt-free spice blend, and ¼ cup of Reuben sauce. Repeat with three more bread slices, then top the four sandwiches with the remaining bread slices and serve.

SHORTCUT: Use ¾ teaspoon of store-bought salt-free spice blend and ¼ teaspoon of nutritional yeast in place of the homemade spice blend.

PER SERVING: Calories: 228; Total fat: 3g; Total carbs: 40g; Fiber: 8g; Sugar: 13g; Protein: 12g; Sodium: 765mg

Vegetable Pita Pizzas

30 MINUTES   EASY PREP   NUT-FREE   SOY-FREE

PREP TIME: 5 minutes   **COOK TIME:** 15 minutes   **SERVES:** 2

This recipe is fun to prep and easily customizable. I always have pita bread and tomato sauce on hand so I can use whatever veggies I have to satisfy my pizza craving or to make a quick dinner on a busy (or lazy) night. The avocado adds a creaminess that is often missed on pizzas without cheese.

4 whole-grain pitas

1 cup Weeknight Tomato Sauce (page 18)

Pinch red pepper flakes (optional)

¼ cup ½-inch broccoli florets

¼ cup shredded spinach

¼ cup chopped asparagus

¼ cup sliced grape tomatoes

¼ cup sliced red onion

¼ cup sliced red bell pepper

¼ cup sliced olives

¼ cup sliced mushrooms

1 avocado, pitted, peeled, and diced

1. Place the whole-grain pitas on a baking sheet in a cold oven and preheat to 350°F. The pitas will warm and the top side should get slightly crispy.

2. Remove the pitas from the oven and flip them over onto a plate, crispy-side down.

3. Spread ¼ cup of tomato sauce on each pita. Add the red pepper flakes (if using).

4. Evenly divide the broccoli, spinach, asparagus, tomatoes, onion, bell pepper, olives, and mushrooms between the pitas.

5. Bake the pizzas for 12 minutes, or until the pita edges are lightly browned and the vegetables are crisp-tender.

6. Divide the avocado between the pitas and serve.

VARIATION TIP: Mix up your toppings! I have added corn, chickpeas, and roasted red peppers.

SHORTCUT: Use your favorite store-bought oil-free tomato or pizza sauce in place of the homemade sauce.

PER SERVING: Calories: 381; Total fat: 19g; Total carbs: 51g; Fiber: 15g; Sugar: 8g; Protein: 11g; Sodium: 402mg

Black Bean and Sweet Potato Tacos

`30 MINUTES` `GLUTEN-FREE` `NUT-FREE` `ONE POT` `SOY-FREE`

PREP TIME: 10 minutes **COOK TIME:** 15 minutes **SERVES:** 4

Protein-packed black beans and luscious sweet potatoes are a terrific way to veganize Taco Tuesday. I love the unique combination of hearty pumpkin seeds and fresh pomegranate seeds. This recipe is a real plant-based winner!

2 teaspoons minced garlic (about 2 cloves)

1 tablespoon water

1 pound sweet potatoes, unpeeled and cut into ½-inch cubes

1 small jalapeño pepper, thinly sliced

1 (15-ounce) can black beans, drained and rinsed

½ teaspoon salt

¼ teaspoon freshly ground black pepper

8 oil-free corn tortillas, warmed according to package instructions

Pumpkin seeds and/or pomegranate seeds, for garnish (optional)

1. In a large skillet over medium-high heat, combine the garlic and water and cook until the garlic is fragrant. Add the sweet potatoes and jalapeño and cook, stirring frequently, for about 10 minutes, until the sweet potatoes are tender. Add 1 to 2 tablespoons of water as needed to prevent burning.

2. Add the beans, salt, and pepper and gently stir together. Cover, reduce the heat to medium, and cook for about 3 minutes, until the beans are just heated through.

3. Scoop the potatoes and beans into the tortillas, sprinkle with pumpkin and/or pomegranate seeds (if using), and serve.

VARIATION TIP: This is delicious as is, but feel free to add your favorite vegan toppings, such as onion, lettuce, or avocado.

PER SERVING: Calories: 311; Total fat: 2g; Total carbs: 64g; Fiber: 13g; Sugar: 5g; Protein: 11g; Sodium: 376mg

VegInspired Plant-Based Bowl Formula

30 MINUTES EASY PREP GLUTEN-FREE NUT-FREE SOY-FREE

PREP TIME: 5 minutes **COOK TIME:** Varies **SERVES:** 2

My plant-based bowl formula is a way for you to add variety and get some inspiration for your own meals. My motto here is "keep it simple." The ingredients in these bowls can be batch-cooked ahead of time and reheated, which brings the meal together super-fast. My favorite VegInspired bowl is made with tricolored quinoa, Savory Braised Tempeh (page 23), baby spinach, raw bell peppers, raw carrot, shredded cabbage, sliced tomatoes, roasted broccoli, Go-To Bowl Sauce (page 16), and 2 tablespoons of walnuts. I encourage you to experiment to find your own favorite combos.

2 cups cooked grains, such as rice, quinoa, farro, or freekeh

1 cup protein, such as beans, tofu, or tempeh

1 cup chopped greens, such as baby spinach, mixed greens, or massaged kale

2 cups raw, roasted, or steamed vegetables of choice

½ cup sauce, such as Go-To Bowl Sauce (page 16)

Optional Toppings

Nuts, such as raw walnut pieces, raw sliced almonds, or roasted unsalted peanuts

Seeds, such as pumpkin seeds, sunflower seeds, hemp hearts, or flaxseed

Seasoned rice vinegar, balsamic vinegar, or red wine vinegar

Olives, pickles, or sauerkraut

1. Evenly divide the grains, protein, greens, and vegetables between two bowls.

2. Top with the sauce and optional toppings (if using). Serve.

PREPARATION TIP: Buy prepped vegetables to bring these bowls together quickly.

SHORTCUT: Use tahini mixed with rice vinegar in place of the Go-To Bowl Sauce.

PER SERVING: Calories: 380; Total fat: 4g; Total carbs: 69g; Fiber: 17g; Sugar: 4g; Protein: 18g; Sodium: 57mg

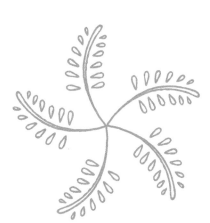

Turmeric Tempeh Stir-Fry

PREP TIME: 10 minutes **COOK TIME:** 20 minutes **SERVES:** 2

Rich and tender marinated tempeh steals the show in this stir-fry. Packed with protein and prebiotics, this often overlooked soy product is a nutritious option for replacing animal protein.

1 tablespoon minced garlic

1 tablespoon unseasoned rice vinegar

1 tablespoon tamari or low-sodium soy sauce

1 teaspoon ground cinnamon

1 teaspoon ground turmeric

1 teaspoon ground cumin

1 teaspoon chili powder

1 (8-ounce) package tempeh, cut into 16 cubes

2 large carrots, diced

1 large red bell pepper, sliced

1 large yellow bell pepper, sliced

6 ounces kale, stemmed and chopped

2 teaspoons arrowroot powder

1. In a medium bowl, combine the garlic, vinegar, tamari, cinnamon, turmeric, cumin, and chili powder and whisk until combined. Add the tempeh and toss to coat. Let sit for 5 minutes.

2. Drain the tempeh, reserving the marinade.

3. In a large skillet or wok over medium heat, cook the tempeh, stirring, for 4 to 6 minutes, until it begins to brown. Add the carrots, red and yellow bell peppers, and kale and cook, stirring, for 3 to 5 minutes, until the kale has brightened in color and the carrots are tender. Add 1 to 2 tablespoons of water as needed to prevent burning.

4. Whisk the arrowroot into the reserved marinade until smooth. Pour the mixture into the skillet, stir to combine, and simmer for 3 minutes more, until thickened.

5. Divide the tempeh mixture between two plates, drizzle with the thickened marinade, and serve.

INGREDIENT TIP: Be sure to use gluten-free tempeh and tamari.

PREPARATION TIP: Let the tempeh marinate in an airtight container overnight or up to 3 days. That extra time makes it incredibly tender!

PER SERVING: Calories: 378; Total fat: 14g; Total carbs: 43g; Fiber: 10g; Sugar: 9g; Protein: 29g; Sodium: 395mg

Tofu Pad Thai

30 MINUTES **GLUTEN-FREE** **NUT-FREE**

PREP TIME: 10 minutes **COOK TIME:** 20 minutes **SERVES:** 4

This quick pad Thai replaces the traditional tamarind sauce for one of lime juice, molasses, and maple syrup for greater ease.

1 (16-ounce) package of brown rice noodles

¼ cup freshly squeezed lime juice

2 tablespoons low-sodium soy sauce

2 tablespoons liquid aminos

1 teaspoon molasses

1 tablespoon pure maple syrup

¾ cup julienned carrots

¾ cup thinly sliced red bell pepper

2 garlic cloves, minced

½ cup 1-inch sliced scallions, green and white parts

1 (14-ounce) package firm tofu, drained

1 cup mung bean sprouts, rinsed

¼ cup unsalted peanuts, chopped (optional)

Chopped fresh cilantro, for garnish (optional)

1 lime, cut into wedges (optional)

1. Submerge the brown rice noodles in hot water and soak for 8 to 10 minutes. Set aside.

2. Meanwhile, in a small bowl, whisk together the lime juice, soy sauce, liquid aminos, molasses, and maple syrup. Set aside.

3. In a large nonstick skillet or sauté pan over medium-high heat, combine the carrots and red bell pepper and cook for 4 to 5 minutes, until soft. Add 1 to 2 tablespoons of water as needed to prevent burning.

4. Add the garlic and scallions and cook for 1 to 2 minutes, until fragrant.

5. Crumble the tofu into the pan, stir to combine, and cook for about 5 minutes, stirring occasionally and adding water to prevent sticking as necessary.

6. Add the sauce mixture, the noodles, and the mung beans and stir to combine. Cook an additional 3 to 5 minutes, until everything is heated through and the sauce has thickened slightly. Serve topped with the peanuts (if using), cilantro (if using), and a lime wedge on the side (if using).

PER SERVING: Calories: 536; Total fat: 5g; Total carbs: 105g; Fiber: 5g; Sugar: 9g; Protein: 17g; Sodium: 494mg

Hawaiian-Inspired Luau Burgers

30 MINUTES   NUT-FREE   SOY-FREE

PREP TIME: 15 minutes   **COOK TIME:** 10 minutes   **SERVES:** 8

Burgers are a staple in my house, especially when I was transitioning to a plant-based life. The combination of black beans, sweet pineapple juice, and barbecue sauce in this recipe comes together for a mouth-watering patty that is ready for grilling anytime. If you are unable to find whole-grain burger buns in your area, try using a whole-grain English muffin instead.

2 (15-ounce) cans black beans, drained and rinsed (or 3 cups cooked black beans)

2 cups cooked brown rice (page 137)

1 cup quick-cooking oats

¼ cup pineapple juice

½ cup Barbecue Sauce (page 19), divided

1 teaspoon garlic powder

1 teaspoon onion powder

1 pineapple, sliced into ¼-inch-thick rings

8 whole-wheat buns

Lettuce, tomato, pickles, and onion, for topping (optional)

1. Preheat the grill to medium-high heat.

2. In a large bowl, use a fork to mash the black beans.

3. Mix in the rice, oats, pineapple juice, ¼ cup of barbecue sauce, the garlic powder, and onion powder. Continue stirring until the mixture begins to hold its shape and can be formed into patties.

4. Scoop out ½ cup of the bean mixture and form it into a patty. Repeat until all of the bean mixture is used.

5. Place the patties on the hot grill and cook for 4 to 5 minutes on each side, flipping once the burgers easily release from the grill surface.

6. After you flip the burgers, place the pineapple rings on the grill and cook for 1 to 2 minutes on each side.

7. Remove the burgers and pineapple rings from the grill. Place one patty and one pineapple ring on each bun along with a spoonful of the remaining barbecue sauce. Top with your favorite burger fixings (if using) and serve.

PREPARATION TIP: If the weather is less than ideal for outdoor cooking, bake the patties on a parchment paper–lined baking sheet at 425°F for 25 to 30 minutes, flipping once halfway through.

SHORTCUT: Use a store-bought oil-free barbecue sauce in place of the homemade barbecue sauce.

PER SERVING: Calories: 422; Total fat: 5g; Total carbs: 83g; Fiber: 12g; Sugar: 21g; Protein: 15g; Sodium: 384mg

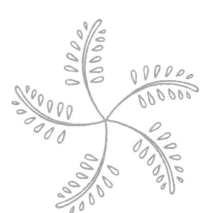

Cajun-Inspired Red Beans and Rice

30 MINUTES **GLUTEN-FREE** **NUT-FREE** **ONE POT** **SOY-FREE**

PREP TIME: 10 minutes   **COOK TIME:** 20 minutes   **SERVES:** 4

Traditional red beans and rice takes hours of simmering and uses animal products. Here we use canned red beans, but feel free to use homecooked beans with 1 cup of bean liquid, if you prefer, and introduce smoked paprika to replace the flavor of the traditional smoky meats. Keeping with Cajun tradition, we use the bell pepper, onion, and celery trinity and add some hot sauce. My chile-head husband insists on serving this with additional hot sauce.

½ cup diced green
   bell pepper
1 cup diced onion
½ cup diced celery
2 to 3 garlic cloves,
   minced (about
   2 tablespoons)
2 tablespoons water
2 (15-ounce) cans
   red beans
1 teaspoon hot sauce
½ teaspoon
   smoked paprika
½ teaspoon salt
½ teaspoon thyme
½ teaspoon freshly
   ground black pepper
1 bay leaf
4 cups cooked rice

1. In a large nonstick skillet or sauté pan over medium-low heat, combine the bell pepper, onion, celery, garlic, and water. Sweat, covered, for about 10 minutes, until softened. Stir occasionally to ensure the mixture does not stick.

2. Add the beans and their liquid, hot sauce, paprika, salt, thyme, pepper, and bay leaf. Stir to combine. Simmer vigorously, uncovered, for 10 minutes, until thickened.

3. Remove and discard the bay leaf. Serve over rice.

PER SERVING: Calories: 410; Total fat: 3g; Total carbs: 81g; Fiber: 15g; Sugar: 3g; Protein: 17g; Sodium: 323mg

Creamy Mushrooms
and Noodles

30 MINUTES

PREP TIME: 10 minutes **COOK TIME:** 15 minutes **SERVES:** 4

This recipe is inspired by creamy beef Stroganoff with plants taking the lead. I use rotini in place of egg noodles, since eggs are not part of a plant-based diet. You could use gluten-free noodles as well. Using a combination of mushrooms and soy sauce brings the necessary umami found in a traditional beef dish. The luscious coconut milk paired with nutritional yeast and chickpea flour creates a thick and buttery sauce.

1 (16-ounce) box whole-grain rotini pasta

8 ounces cremini mushrooms, sliced

1 medium shallot, finely diced (about 2 tablespoons)

1 tablespoon low-sodium soy sauce

1 (15-ounce) can lite coconut milk

2 tablespoons nutritional yeast

1 tablespoon chickpea flour

¼ teaspoon salt

¼ teaspoon freshly ground black pepper

1. Bring a large pot of water to a boil over high heat. Add the pasta and cook according to package instructions until tender, usually about 10 minutes, then drain.

2. Meanwhile, in a large sauté pan or skillet over medium heat, add the mushrooms and shallots and cook, stirring frequently, for about 5 to 7 minutes, until the mushrooms are bright and glistening. Add 1 to 2 tablespoons of water as needed to prevent burning.

3. Add the soy sauce, coconut milk, nutritional yeast, chickpea flour, salt, and pepper and stir to combine. Simmer for 3 to 5 minutes, until the sauce has thickened.

4. Stir the mushroom mixture into the noodles and serve warm.

PER SERVING: Calories: 514; Total fat: 12g; Total carbs: 90g; Fiber: 10g; Sugar: 1g; Protein: 20g; Sodium: 292mg

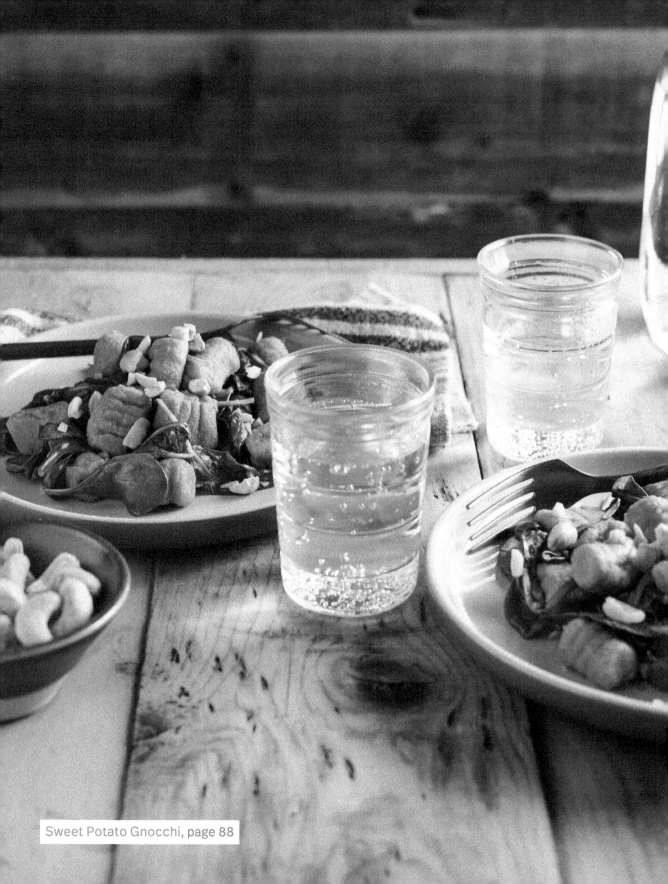

Sweet Potato Gnocchi, page 88

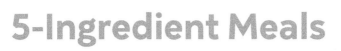

5-Ingredient Meals

Savory Avocado Toast

PREP TIME: 5 minutes **SERVES:** 1

Using a whole-grain bread for your avocado toast gives you a nice serving of heart-healthy fiber. The combination of mashed avocado, lemon juice, and the salt-free spice blend is a party for your mouth, but adding roasted red peppers really amps up the celebration. Be sure to choose oil-free red peppers.

1 avocado, pitted and peeled

2 whole-grain bread slices, toasted

6 tablespoons oil-free roasted red pepper, sliced

1 teaspoon freshly squeezed lemon juice

2 teaspoons Salt-Free Spice Blend (page 14)

1. Mash half of the avocado on each slice of toast.

2. Evenly divide the red pepper between the slices of toast. Drizzle on ½ teaspoon of lemon juice per slice, and sprinkle with 1 teaspoon of the salt-free spice blend. Serve right away.

SHORTCUT: Use 1½ teaspoons of store-bought salt-free spice blend plus ½ teaspoon of nutritional yeast in place of the homemade version.

VARIATION TIP: Adding a pinch of red pepper flakes or a drizzle of sriracha satisfies a spicy craving.

PER SERVING: Calories: 503; Total fat: 32g; Total carbs: 49g; Fiber: 18g; Sugar: 7g; Protein: 13g; Sodium: 307mg

Barbecue Beans on Toast

5 INGREDIENT **30 MINUTES** **EASY PREP** **NUT-FREE** **ONE POT** **SOY-FREE**

PREP TIME: 5 minutes **COOK TIME:** 10 minutes **SERVES:** 2

Inspired by English beans on toast, I set out to make a savory, satisfying breakfast—and this is a winner. The tangy sauce that coats the beans adds a zing of flavor to an otherwise boring piece of toast. It's a "right proper" breakfast on its own or as an accompaniment to the Sheet Pan Scrambled Tofu and Potatoes (page 96).

1 (15-ounce) can navy
   beans, drained
   and rinsed

½ cup Barbecue Sauce
   (page 19)

1 tablespoon vegan
   Worcestershire sauce

¼ teaspoon garlic powder

4 whole-grain bread
   slices, toasted

1. In a small saucepan over medium heat, combine the beans, barbecue sauce, Worcestershire sauce, and garlic powder. Simmer for 5 to 7 minutes, until heated through.

2. Scoop ½ cup of the bean mixture onto a slice toasted bread. Continue with remaining mixture and toast. Serve warm.

INGREDIENT TIP: You can find nut-free, gluten-free, and soy-free versions of vegan Worcestershire sauce, but be sure to read the label—they sometimes contain coconut and/or soy.

SHORTCUT: Use an oil-free store-bought barbecue sauce in place of homemade.

PER SERVING: Calories: 422; Total fat: 3g; Total carbs: 79g; Fiber: 19g; Sugar: 16g; Protein: 20g; Sodium: 642mg

Maple-Pecan Granola

5 INGREDIENT **EASY PREP** **GLUTEN-FREE** **SOY-FREE**

PREP TIME: 5 minutes, plus 30 minutes to cool **COOK TIME:** 20 minutes **SERVES:** 4

I enjoy having homemade, crunchy granola on hand for an instant snack or to add to plant-based milk like a bowl of cereal. Making your own granola allows you to control the ingredients.

1½ cups rolled oats

¼ cup pecan pieces

¼ cup pure maple syrup

1 teaspoon vanilla extract

½ teaspoon ground cinnamon

1. Preheat the oven to 300°F. Line a baking sheet with parchment paper.

2. In a large bowl, combine the oats, pecans, maple syrup, vanilla extract, and cinnamon. Stir until the oats and pecans are completely coated.

3. Spread the mixture on the baking sheet in an even layer. Bake for 20 minutes, stirring once after 10 minutes.

4. Remove from the oven and allow to cool on the countertop for 30 minutes before serving. The granola may still be a bit soft right after you remove it from the oven, but it will gradually firm up as it cools.

VARIATION TIP: Once the granola has cooled, add in some of your favorite dried fruits to make a tasty trail mix.

PER SERVING: Calories: 254; Total fat: 8g; Total carbs: 40g; Fiber: 5g; Sugar: 12g; Protein: 7g; Sodium: 4mg

Berry Oat Bowl

PREP TIME: 30 minutes **SERVES:** 1

This is an excellent make-and-take breakfast. I love the texture of these slightly softened oats after letting them sit for 30 minutes, but honestly, these oats can be eaten right away if you don't feel like waiting. Just layer the ingredients and pour the milk over them like you would any cereal.

½ cup rolled oats

½ cup unsweetened plant-based milk

½ cup sliced fresh berries

1 tablespoon pure maple syrup

⅛ teaspoon vanilla extract

1. In a bowl with a lid, mix together the oats, milk, berries, maple syrup, and vanilla.

2. Set aside for 15 to 30 minutes, until the oats have softened slightly, then enjoy.

PER SERVING: Calories: 310; Total fat: 5g; Total carbs: 57g; Fiber: 7g; Sugar: 20g; Protein: 10g; Sodium: 63mg

Potato Breakfast Skillet

5 INGREDIENT **GLUTEN-FREE** **NUT-FREE** **ONE POT** **SOY-FREE**

PREP TIME: 10 minutes **COOK TIME:** 25 minutes **SERVES:** 2

I can't pass up a good potato dish, and this one does not disappoint! Simple and ready in about 35 minutes, this starchy breakfast is a great weekday meal. Try it topped with ketchup, or change it up by using sweet potatoes instead of regular potatoes. Just simmer for a little less time, checking them after 10 minutes to make sure they don't go mushy.

1 cup diced onion

½ cup diced bell pepper (any color)

4 cups diced yellow or red potatoes

1 cup vegetable broth

1 tablespoon Salt-Free Spice Blend (page 14)

1 cup loosely packed baby spinach

1. In a large nonstick sauté pan or skillet, combine the onion and bell pepper and cook, stirring, for 3 to 5 minutes, until they start to soften. Add 1 to 2 tablespoons of water as needed to prevent burning.

2. Add the potatoes, broth, and salt-free blend, stirring to combine. Cover and simmer for 10 to 15 minutes.

3. Add the spinach and continue to simmer, covered, for 5 minutes, or until the potatoes are knife-tender. Serve hot.

SHORTCUT: Use a store-bought salt-free spice blend plus 1 teaspoon of nutritional yeast in place of the homemade version.

PER SERVING: Calories: 257; Total fat: 1g; Total carbs: 58g; Fiber: 8g; Sugar: 9g; Protein: 7g; Sodium: 71mg

Waffle and Fruit Skewers

5 INGREDIENT **30 MINUTES** **NUT-FREE**

PREP TIME: 10 minutes **COOK TIME:** 10 minutes **SERVES:** 2

Having fun with food is always encouraged in my house, and this super-simple recipe will soon become a favorite in yours. I use store-bought waffles, but homecooked ones or even Plant-Powered Pancakes (page 48) could be used for a less-processed option. Although a subtle accompaniment, the tahini sauces really steal the show, so don't skip out!

For the tahini-jam sauce

2 tablespoons tahini

2 tablespoons low-sugar or sugar-free jam of your choice

1 tablespoon water

For the skewers

4 oil-free whole-grain vegan waffles, such as Food For Life Ezekiel brand

1 cup sliced strawberries

1 cup orange or clementine segments

1. **Make the tahini-jam sauce:** In a separate small bowl, whisk together the tahini, jam, and water.

2. **Make the skewers:** Cook the waffles according to package instructions, usually by toasting for about 5 minutes. Cut them into quarters.

3. Alternate placing waffle pieces and fruit on wooden or metal skewers until all of the ingredients are used up. Plate the skewers.

4. Drizzle with the sauce and serve.

VARIATION TIP: For a sweet and tart sauce, substitute lemon juice for the water. For a jam-free option, make a maple-tahini sauce by whisking together 2 tablespoons of tahini, 2 tablespoons of maple syrup, 1 tablespoon of lemon juice, ⅛ teaspoon of ground cinnamon.

PER SERVING: Calories: 763; Total fat: 37g; Total carbs: 94g; Fiber: 9g; Sugar: 30g; Protein: 18g; Sodium: 805mg

Chocolate and Peanut Butter Quinoa

5 INGREDIENT **30 MINUTES** **EASY PREP** **GLUTEN-FREE** **ONE POT** **SOY-FREE**

PREP TIME: 5 minutes **COOK TIME:** 10 minutes **SERVES:** 2

Is there a better pair than chocolate and peanut butter? I think not! I could eat this dessert-like meal any time of day, and since the quinoa provides a nice serving of protein, it satisfies my hunger, too. Peanut powder comes in handy for this recipe because it easily mixes with the other ingredients and adds less fat; if you substitute regular peanut butter, your nutritional information will vary from what is listed here.

1 cup unsweetened
plant-based milk

2 cups cooked quinoa
(page 137)

1 tablespoon pure
maple syrup

1 tablespoon unsweet-
ened cocoa powder

1 tablespoon defatted
peanut powder

1. In a medium saucepan over medium-high heat, bring the milk to a boil, then immediately reduce the heat to low.

2. Stir in the quinoa, maple syrup, cocoa powder, and peanut powder. Cook, uncovered, for 5 minutes, stirring every other minute. Serve warm.

VARIATION TIP: The recipe calls for 1 tablespoon of maple syrup, but if you would like it sweeter you can always add in a bit more or top the quinoa with a sliced banana.

PER SERVING: Calories: 330; Total fat: 7g; Total carbs: 53g; Fiber: 7g; Sugar: 11g; Protein: 14g; Sodium: 90mg

Carrot Soup

5 INGREDIENT **30 MINUTES** **EASY PREP** **GLUTEN-FREE** **NUT-FREE**

PREP TIME: 5 minutes **COOK TIME:** 20 minutes **SERVES:** 4

Sweet carrots harmonize with bright dill in this brothy soup, hitting just the right notes to leave you wanting a second bowl. I prefer to use fresh organic carrots in this recipe simply because I find them to be a bit sweeter, which yields a tastier soup.

4 cups chopped organic carrots

4 tablespoons Salt-Free Spice Blend (page 14)

2 tablespoons dried dill

2 teaspoons ground cumin

4 cups vegetable broth

2 teaspoons red miso paste

¼ teaspoon freshly ground black pepper

1. In a large saucepan or Dutch oven over medium heat, place the carrots and cook, stirring, for 1 to 2 minutes. Add 1 to 2 tablespoons of water as needed to prevent burning.

2. Add the salt-free spice blend, dill, and cumin. Sauté for 1 to 2 minutes, until fragrant.

3. Add the broth. Increase the heat to medium high and bring to a boil, then reduce the heat to medium-low. Simmer, partially covered, for 15 minutes, until the carrots are tender.

4. In a high-speed blender (or using an immersion blender), blend the carrots with 1 cup of cooking broth until smooth. Add the carrot mixture back to the pan. Add the miso and stir to combine. Season with the pepper and serve.

SHORTCUT: Use 3 tablespoons of a store-bought salt-free spice blend plus 1 tablespoon of nutritional yeast in place of the homemade version.

PER SERVING: Calories: 77; Total fat: 1g; Total carbs: 16g; Fiber: 4g; Sugar: 8g; Protein: 2g; Sodium: 186mg

Lime-Mint Soup

5 INGREDIENT 30 MINUTES EASY PREP GLUTEN-FREE NUT-FREE ONE POT
SOY-FREE

PREP TIME: 5 minutes **COOK TIME:** 20 minutes **SERVES:** 4

This soup has lifted my mood and satisfied my palate on many a cold night. It is great for sipping as a hot broth during the winter months, but it is best enjoyed over a bed of freshly cooked brown jasmine rice or quinoa.

4 cups vegetable broth

¼ cup coarsely chopped fresh mint leaves

¼ cup chopped scallions, green and white parts

3 garlic cloves, minced

3 tablespoons freshly squeezed lime juice

1. In a large stock pot over medium-high heat, combine the broth, mint, scallions, garlic, and lime juice. Bring to a boil, then reduce the heat to low.

2. Cover and simmer for 15 minutes, until the flavors have melded. Serve hot.

INGREDIENT TIP: When selecting mint leaves, look for brightly colored, unblemished leaves.

PER SERVING: Calories: 22; Total fat: 0g; Total carbs: 6g; Fiber: 1g; Sugar: 2g; Protein: 0g; Sodium: 54mg

Creamy Basil-Tomato Soup

5 INGREDIENT 30 MINUTES EASY PREP FREEZES WELL GLUTEN-FREE NUT-FREE

ONE POT SOY-FREE

PREP TIME: 5 minutes **COOK TIME:** 20 minutes **SERVES:** 4

As I simmered a batch of tomato sauce one day, I had a craving for creamy tomato soup. Remembering something I had scrolled past on Pinterest, I pulled out a can of lite coconut milk and added it to my sauce. With a little nutritional yeast and black pepper, I had creamy tomato soup in minutes! It really doesn't get much easier than that.

2 batches Weeknight
  Tomato Sauce (page 18)

1 (15-ounce) can lite
  coconut milk

1 tablespoon nutritional
  yeast

¼ teaspoon freshly
  ground black pepper

1. In a medium saucepan over medium heat, stir together the tomato sauce, coconut milk, nutritional yeast, and pepper. Bring to a simmer, then cook for 10 to 15 minutes, until the soup is fragrant and heated through.

2. Serve warm.

SHORTCUT: Use store-bought oil-free pasta sauce and 1 cup of fresh basil in place of homemade sauce.

PER SERVING: Calories: 81; Total fat: 4g; Total carbs: 9g; Fiber: 2g; Sugar: 4g; Protein: 2g; Sodium: 258mg

Barbecue Cauliflower Tacos

5 INGREDIENT **EASY PREP** **GLUTEN-FREE** **NUT-FREE** **SOY-FREE**

PREP TIME: 5 minutes **COOK TIME:** 30 minutes **SERVES:** 2

Tacos always remind me of snacking, and I am a snack lover at heart. Roasted cauliflower makes for a distinct, smoky, and veggie-friendly snack or meal. Baking your cauliflower tossed in the barbecue sauce creates a caramelized sauce, but if you prefer a fresher option, you can also toss your roasted cauliflower after baking.

1 head cauliflower, cut into 1-inch florets

1 cup Barbecue Sauce (page 19)

6 oil-free corn or whole-grain tortillas

1 avocado, pitted, peeled, and sliced

1 lime, cut into 6 wedges

1. Preheat the oven to 425°F.

2. In a large bowl, toss the cauliflower with the barbecue sauce. Transfer to a parchment-lined baking sheet.

3. Bake the cauliflower for 30 minutes, until the cauliflower is tender and the barbecue sauce has started to caramelize.

4. Meanwhile, warm the tortillas according to the package instructions and place them in a tea towel to keep them warm and pliable.

5. On top of each tortilla, layer the barbecue cauliflower bites, two pieces of sliced avocado, and a squeeze of lime. Serve.

SHORTCUT: Use an oil-free store-bought barbecue sauce in place of the homemade version.

VARIATION TIP: Optional additional toppings include shredded cabbage, rinsed sliced onions, and chopped fresh cilantro.

PER SERVING: Calories: 536; Total fat: 18g; Total carbs: 90g; Fiber: 17g; Sugar: 31g; Protein: 13g; Sodium: 421mg

Avocado Sushi

5 INGREDIENT **GLUTEN-FREE** **NO COOK** **NUT-FREE** **SOY-FREE**

PREP TIME: 10 minutes, plus 30 minutes to chill **SERVES:** 4

I wasn't introduced to sushi until I was an adult and living on my own, but I quickly found it to be something I enjoyed. I am thrilled that I can continue to enjoy a vegetable version such as this one. I like to use short-grain brown rice as it more resembles sushi rice.

½ cup cold cooked brown rice (page 137)

1 tablespoon mirin or rice vinegar

1 large date, pitted and finely chopped

1 large avocado, halved and pitted

4 (8-by-7-inch) nori sheets

1. In a medium bowl, mix together the rice, mirin, and dates. Refrigerate for at least 30 minutes.

2. Using the tip of a sharp knife, cut each avocado half into four slices. Using a spoon, gently scoop the slices out of the peel and set them aside on a small plate.

3. Place one sheet of nori on a cutting board. Spoon 1 tablespoon of the chilled brown rice mixture onto the nori, making a line of rice on the edge closest to you. Add two avocado slices on top of the rice.

4. Lift the edge of the nori sheet that is furthest from you away from the cutting board and tightly roll it over the filling toward you, using your thumbs to keep the filling inside, until the filling is completely enclosed. Repeat with the remaining ingredients to create four rolls.

5. Serve the rolls whole, or cut each into four pieces.

VARIATION TIP: Carrot, cucumber, and bell pepper sticks are all great substitutes for avocado—just be careful not to overfill the nori or it will be hard to roll. Pick just one!

PER SERVING: Calories: 132; Total fat: 8g; Total carbs: 15g; Fiber: 5g; Sugar: 5g; Protein: 2g; Sodium: 97mg

Tofu Fried Rice

5 INGREDIENT   30 MINUTES   EASY PREP   GLUTEN-FREE   NUT-FREE   ONE POT

PREP TIME: 5 minutes **COOK TIME:** 15 minutes **SERVES:** 4

Faster than takeout, oil-free, and delicious, this fried rice is a week-night winner! Keeping a batch of cooked brown rice (page 137) in your refrigerator and vegetables in your freezer for meals like this is highly recommended to keep things simple. It thrills me that this meal can satisfy my craving for takeout and align with my plant-based eating goals.

1 (14-ounce) block firm
   tofu, drained and
   crumbled

1 cup frozen carrots

2 cups frozen stir-fry
   vegetables

2 tablespoons water

3 cups cooked brown rice
   (page 137)

¼ cup tamari or
   low-sodium soy sauce

1. In a large nonstick skillet over medium-low heat, combine the tofu, carrots, vegetables, and water. Cook, stirring occasionally, for about 5 minutes, or until the vegetables are softened.

2. Add the rice and tamari and stir to combine.

3. Cook for 5 to 7 minutes, until the rice is warmed and heated through. Serve warm.

INGREDIENT TIP: I like to use a stir-fry blend because it often has both mushrooms and onions, but feel free to mix and match your own vegetables. Frozen asparagus or cut green beans are also great alternatives. You can always add sliced scallions if your vegetable blend excludes onions.

PER SERVING: Calories: 320; Total fat: 6g; Total carbs: 51g; Fiber: 9g; Sugar: 6g; Protein: 17g; Sodium: 648mg

Vegetable Hummus Pasta

5 INGREDIENT **30 MINUTES** **EASY PREP** **NUT-FREE** **ONE POT** **SOY-FREE**

PREP TIME: 5 minutes **COOK TIME:** 20 minutes **SERVES:** 4

My mind is still blown about how uncomplicated yet yummy this recipe is. I love being able to cook my frozen vegetables with my pasta and drain them together. It makes this an easy one-pot meal and ready in minutes. I use a plain hummus, but roasted red pepper or another flavor would add a fancier flair.

4 quarts water

1 (16-ounce) box whole-grain shell pasta

1 (10-ounce) bag frozen cauliflower, broccoli, and carrot blend

1 cup oil-free hummus

½ cup sliced kalamata olives

1 tablespoon Salt-Free Spice Blend (page 14)

1. In a large saucepan over high heat, bring the water to a boil. Add the pasta and cook for 2 minutes less than the package instructions indicate, usually 6 to 8 minutes.

2. Add frozen vegetables to the pot with the pasta and cook for another 6 to 8 minutes, or until pasta is tender.

3. Reserve 1 cup of cooking water, then drain the pasta and vegetables and return them to the saucepan.

4. Add the hummus, olives, and salt-free spice blend. Add the reserved cooking water, a little at a time, and stir until you have a creamy sauce. Serve warm.

PREPARATION TIP: Be sure to reserve the pasta water to use, which makes your pasta creamy. You can add any remaining pasta water to the pasta dish before storing leftovers to keep them creamy.

SHORTCUT: Use a store-bought salt-free spice blend plus 1 teaspoon of nutritional yeast in place of the homemade version.

PER SERVING: Calories: 498; Total fat: 5g; Total carbs: 100g; Fiber: 15g; Sugar: 4g; Protein: 22g; Sodium: 152mg

Tahini and Curry Cauliflower

5 INGREDIENT · 30 MINUTES · EASY PREP · GLUTEN-FREE · NUT-FREE · SOY-FREE

PREP TIME: 5 minutes **COOK TIME:** 20 minutes **SERVES:** 4

This dish is heavenly! The tahini offers a light and airy mouthfeel, while curry brings a warm, earthy flavor. Tahini has always been a secret ingredient in my baking recipes for its creamy texture, and it works just as well in savory dishes.

½ cup tahini

½ cup vegetable broth

1 teaspoon curry powder

¼ teaspoon ground ginger

1 head cauliflower, cut into 1-inch florets

¼ teaspoon freshly ground black pepper

⅛ teaspoon salt

1. Preheat the oven to 400° F and line a baking sheet with parchment paper.

2. In a large bowl, mix together the tahini, broth, curry powder, and ginger until well combined. Add the cauliflower and toss to coat well.

3. Transfer the cauliflower to the prepared baking sheet and spread out into a single layer. Season with the pepper and salt.

4. Bake for 20 minutes, or until the cauliflower is crisp-tender and golden brown. Serve warm.

PER SERVING: Calories: 217; Total fat: 17g; Total carbs: 14g; Fiber: 6g; Sugar: 3g; Protein: 8g; Sodium: 157mg

Pasta and Greens Dinner

5 INGREDIENT | **30 MINUTES** | **EASY PREP** | **NUT-FREE** | **SOY-FREE**

PREP TIME: 5 minutes **COOK TIME:** 20 minutes **SERVES:** 4

As a child, spaghetti dinner was my favorite meal. I created this simple meal one day when I needed to use up some wilting spinach, and I love it! Adding spinach to a store-bought pasta sauce also helps you check off a serving of greens without having to wash a salad bowl. Win-win!

1 (16-ounce) box whole-grain pasta of choice

2 batches Weeknight Tomato Sauce (page 18)

1 (5-ounce) container baby spinach

¼ cup nutritional yeast

1. Bring a large pot of water to a boil over high heat. Add the pasta and cook according to package instructions until tender, usually about 8 minutes. Drain.

2. Meanwhile, in a large saucepan over medium heat, combine the tomato sauce and spinach and stir well. Simmer, stirring occasionally, for about 10 minutes, until the sauce is heated through and the spinach is wilted.

3. Transfer the pasta to the saucepan and mix thoroughly. Serve plated with 1 tablespoon of nutritional yeast sprinkled on top.

SHORTCUT: Use store-bought oil-free pasta sauce in place of the homemade sauce.

VARIATION TIP: To jazz up this dish, stir in 1 (15-ounce) can of white beans, drained and rinsed, to the pot of sauce just before you mix in the pasta.

PER SERVING: Calories: 497; Total fat: 5g; Total carbs: 92g; Fiber: 9g; Sugar: 8g; Protein: 23g; Sodium: 592mg

Tuscan-Inspired Farro Casserole

5 INGREDIENT EASY PREP NUT-FREE ONE POT SOY-FREE

PREP TIME: 5 minutes **COOK TIME:** 1 hour 30 minutes **SERVES:** 2 to 4

One pot and easy to prep, this wholesome farro casserole is an old faithful recipe. The long baking time yields superbly chewy farro with that cooked-all-day texture. Farro is an ancient wheat grain traditionally used in Italian cooking. If you substitute a gluten-free grain, like rice or quinoa, adjust the cooking times accordingly.

2 cups water or
  vegetable broth
1 cup pearled farro
1 (15-ounce) can crushed
  tomatoes
1 (15-ounce) can navy
  beans, drained
1 cup packed
  baby spinach
½ teaspoon garlic powder
½ teaspoon salt
¼ teaspoon freshly
  ground black pepper

1. Preheat the oven to 350°F.

2. In a 2-quart casserole dish with a lid, stir together the water, farro, tomatoes, beans, spinach, garlic powder, salt, and pepper.

3. Bake for 75 to 90 minutes, until the farro is tender. Serve warm.

PER SERVING: Calories: 309; Total fat: 2g; Total carbs: 65g; Fiber: 17g; Sugar: 5g; Protein: 13g; Sodium: 433mg

No-Bake Black Bean and Avocado Enchiladas

5 INGREDIENT   30 MINUTES   EASY PREP   GLUTEN-FREE   NUT-FREE   SOY-FREE

PREP TIME: 5 minutes   **COOK TIME:** 10 minutes   **SERVES:** 2

These enticing enchiladas were inspired by an avocado enchilada I had at a Tex-Mex restaurant. I added beans for a little protein and heartiness, and I simplified the process by taking out the baking step and layering the ingredients versus rolling them. The result was a delicious plate of enchiladas that has become a staple in my house.

8 oil-free corn tortillas

1 (15-ounce) can oil-free enchilada sauce

1 (15-ounce) can black beans, drained and rinsed

2 avocados, pitted, peeled, and sliced

1. Warm the tortillas according to the package instructions and wrap them in a tea towel to keep them warm and pliable.

2. In a small saucepan over medium heat, bring the enchilada sauce to a simmer. Cook, stirring occasionally, for 8 to 10 minutes, until warmed through and fragrant.

3. Starting with one tortilla, dip it in the enchilada sauce and place on a serving plate. Top with 3 tablespoons of beans, half of an avocado's worth of slices,, and another dipped tortilla. Repeat to create a second and third layer (using 4 tortillas), then create a second enchilada in the same way. Serve warm.

INGREDIENT TIP: Be sure to check the label on the can of enchilada sauce. There are oil-free and allergen-free versions, but many brands contain oil, soy, and wheat.

PER SERVING: Calories: 773; Total fat: 33g; Total carbs: 104g; Fiber: 32g; Sugar: 4g; Protein: 23g; Sodium: 747mg

Sweet Potato Gnocchi

5 INGREDIENT   SOY-FREE

PREP TIME: 50 minutes   **COOK TIME:** 20 minutes   **SERVES:** 2

This tasty pasta-inspired dish is worth every minute of rolling and clean up, since you are rewarded with little pockets of sweet potato love. If you are eating this on its own, it will provide two satisfying servings. If you add a protein, like beans, tofu, or lentils, you can stretch the gnocchi to feed more.

1 large sweet potato

¾ cup whole-wheat flour, plus more for the work surface

4 quarts, plus 1 tablespoon water

3 garlic cloves, minced

2 handfuls fresh spinach

1 teaspoon crushed raw cashews

1. Using a fork or the tip of a knife, poke holes in the skin of the sweet potato. Microwave on high power, with the skin on, for 10 minutes, until the flesh is soft.

2. Halve the potato lengthwise and scoop the flesh into a bowl. Mash well using a fork. Add the flour and mix with the fork to combine.

3. Lightly dust a work surface with flour, then transfer the dough to it. Knead for 2 to 3 minutes. Roll the dough into a ½-inch-thick rope. Cut the rope into ¼-inch pieces. Lightly roll the tines of a fork across each piece to create grooves.

4. Meanwhile, bring 4 quarts of water to a boil over high heat, then reduce the heat to medium-low to maintain a simmer (you may need to adjust the heat further). Carefully place the gnocchi in the water. Cook for about 2 minutes, or until they float.

5. In a medium skillet over medium-high heat, heat the remaining 1 tablespoon of water. Add the garlic and sauté for 1 minute. Add the spinach and cook, stirring, for about 2 minutes, until it wilts. Add the cooked gnocchi and cook, stirring, for 1 minute more. Remove from the heat, sprinkle with the cashews, and serve.

PREPARATION TIP: If you don't want to microwave, you can also bake the sweet potato in a 350° F oven for about 1 hour, until soft.

VARIATION TIP: Gnocchi also tastes great with a drizzle of balsamic glaze or a simple dressing made with 2 tablespoons of freshly squeezed lemon juice, 1 teaspoon of grated peeled fresh ginger, and ½ teaspoon of ground cumin.

PER SERVING: Calories: 245; Total fat: 2g; Total carbs: 53g; Fiber: 8g; Sugar: 3g; Protein: 9g; Sodium: 61mg

Chana Masala

5 INGREDIENT **30 MINUTES** **EASY PREP** **GLUTEN-FREE** **NUT-FREE** **ONE POT**
SOY-FREE

PREP TIME: 5 minutes **COOK TIME:** 20 minutes **SERVES:** 6

The headliner in this dish is the warming, sophisticated spice of garam masala. And blending a half cup of chickpeas adds a thick consistency to this dish without affecting the flavor or adding a high-fat option, like coconut milk. I like to serve this with cooked brown rice.

1 onion, sliced

1 small jalapeño or serrano pepper, seeded and minced

2 teaspoons garam masala

1 teaspoon salt

1 teaspoon freshly ground black pepper

1 (14.5-ounce) can roasted-garlic or plain diced tomatoes

2 (15-ounce) cans chickpeas, drained but not rinsed, divided

1. In a large saucepan over medium-high heat, combine the onion and jalapeño. Sauté for about 3 minutes, until the onion softens. Add 1 to 2 tablespoons of water as needed to prevent burning.

2. Add the garam masala, salt, and pepper and sauté for 2 minutes more.

3. Stir in the tomatoes and ½ cup of the chickpeas.

4. Use an immersion blender to roughly puree the mixture in the pan. You're looking for a thick, chunky, salsa-like texture. Alternatively, use a potato masher to mash the mixture in the pan.

5. Add the remainder of the chickpeas and bring to a boil. Reduce the heat to low and simmer, stirring occasionally, for 10 minutes. Add water, if necessary, to maintain a stew-like consistency. Serve warm.

INGREDIENT TIP: If you don't have garam masala on hand, a one-ingredient swap is curry powder. If you're willing to go with two spices, opt for 1 teaspoon each of ground allspice and cumin.

PER SERVING: Calories: 124; Total fat: 2g; Total carbs: 22g; Fiber: 7g; Sugar: 6g; Protein: 6g; Sodium: 628mg

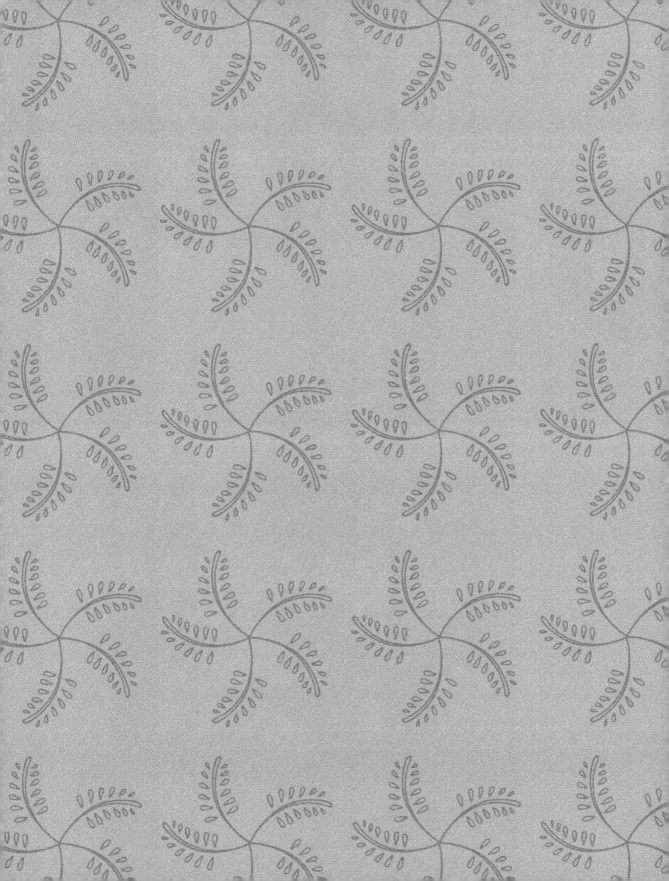

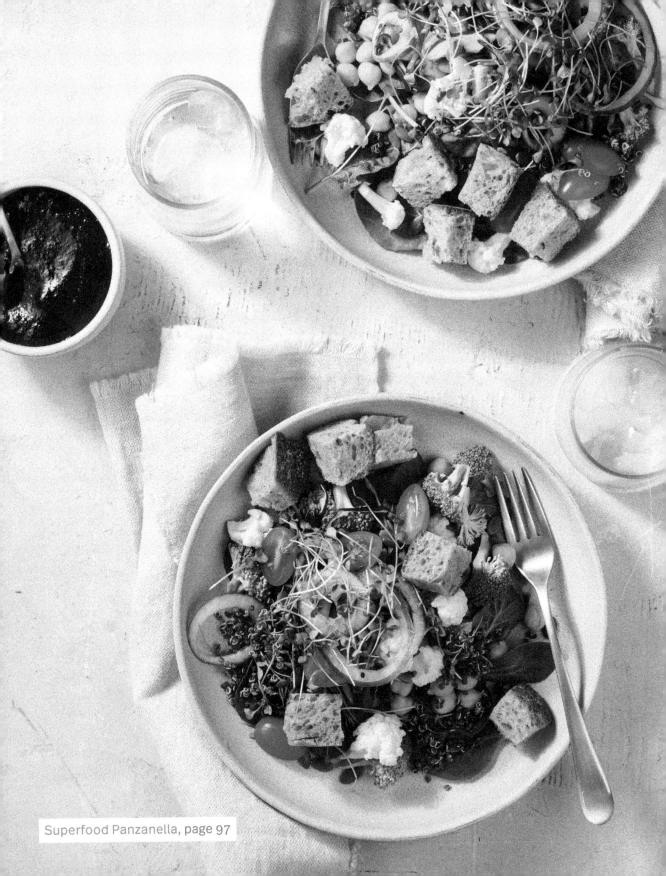

Superfood Panzanella, page 97

CHAPTER 6

One-Pot Meals

Oatmeal Raisin Bowl

EASY PREP **GLUTEN-FREE** **ONE POT** **SOY-FREE**

PREP TIME: 5 minutes **COOK TIME:** 30 minutes **SERVES:** 4

I love steel-cut oats as an alternative to rolled oats. Steel-cut oats are a less processed oat product, and they have a nuttier and chewier texture. Their texture holds up against cooking, and they are packed with fiber, which means they will keep you full for longer and support heart health!

1 cup steel-cut oats

2 cups unsweetened plant-based milk

½ cup unsweetened raisins

1 teaspoon ground cinnamon

¼ cup chopped pitted dates

¼ cup chopped pecans

1. In a large saucepan over medium-high heat, combine the oats, milk, raisins, and cinnamon, and bring to a boil.

2. Reduce the heat to low and simmer, stirring occasionally, for about 25 minutes, until the oats are tender.

3. Remove from the heat. Stir in the dates and pecans, then serve.

INGREDIENT TIP: The dates provide just enough sweetness to omit the need for any additional sugar. If you want to skip the dates, any dried fruit will do—I'm partial to dried cherries sweetened with apple juice. Or try cacao nibs or shredded coconut for a different flavor.

VARIATION TIP: To make this nut-free, omit the pecans and try sunflower seeds instead.

PER SERVING: Calories: 349; Total fat: 10g; Total carbs: 59g; Fiber: 8g; Sugar: 21g; Protein: 10g; Sodium: 62mg

Savory Breakfast Oats

5 INGREDIENT   30 MINUTES   EASY PREP   GLUTEN-FREE   NUT-FREE   ONE POT
SOY-FREE

PREP TIME: 5 minutes   **COOK TIME:** 15 minutes   **SERVES:** 2

I had always thought of oats as a sweet breakfast, but I was inspired by the craze of savory oats, and this dish has become one of my favorite breakfasts. They are delectable as is; however, I love to top them with salty tempeh bacon. You can also start the recipe by sautéing some diced vegetables, so it almost becomes an oat pilaf.

2 cups vegetable broth

1 cup rolled oats

1 cup chickpeas, drained
   and rinsed

1 cup shredded kale

1 tablespoon nutritional
   yeast

1 tablespoon Salt-Free
   Spice Blend (page 14)

1. In a small saucepan over medium-high heat, bring the broth to a boil.

2. Add the oats, chickpeas, kale, nutritional yeast, and salt-free spice blend. Reduce the heat to medium and simmer for 5 to 7 minutes, until oats are tender and start to thicken.

3. Remove from heat and let stand for 5 minutes before serving.

SHORTCUT: In a pinch, use a store-bought salt-free spice blend in place of the homemade version.

PER SERVING: Calories: 301; Total fat: 5g; Total carbs: 54g; Fiber: 8g; Sugar: 6g; Protein: 11g; Sodium: 164mg

Sheet Pan Scrambled Tofu and Potatoes

5 INGREDIENT GLUTEN-FREE NUT-FREE ONE POT

PREP TIME: 10 minutes **COOK TIME:** 35 minutes **SERVES:** 4

Scrambled tofu with potatoes is one of my top breakfasts, but there are days when standing over the stove just doesn't fit into my plan. So I tried tossing everything on a baking sheet and letting the oven do the work, and it was a hit.

10 ounces shredded russet potatoes

1 (14-ounce) block firm tofu, drained

1 tablespoon Salt-Free Spice Blend (page 14)

1 teaspoon onion powder

½ teaspoon freshly ground black pepper

¼ teaspoon garlic powder

¼ teaspoon salt

⅛ teaspoon turmeric

1. Preheat the oven to 400°F and line a baking sheet with parchment paper.

2. Add the shredded potatoes to one side of the pan and crumble the tofu on the other side.

3. Sprinkle half of the salt-free spice blend, onion powder, pepper, garlic powder, salt, and turmeric over the potatoes, then toss or stir them to coat well. Sprinkle the other half of the seasonings over tofu, then toss or stir it to coat well.

4. Bake for 15 minutes, stir, and bake another 15 to 20 minutes, until the tofu is starting to turn a light golden brown and the potatoes are tender and starting to and crisp up. Serve warm.

INGREDIENT TIP: If you want to grate your own potatoes, rinse half of the batch under cool water to remove some of the starch, so the potatoes have a light and airy texture.

SHORTCUT: Use a store-bought salt-free spice blend plus 1 teaspoon of nutritional yeast in place of the homemade version.

PER SERVING: Calories: 129; Total fat: 4g; Total carbs: 15g; Fiber: 2g; Sugar: 1g; Protein: 10g; Sodium: 162mg

Superfood Panzanella

30 MINUTES | **NUT-FREE** | **ONE POT** | **SOY-FREE**

PREP TIME: 15 minutes **COOK TIME:** 5 minutes **SERVES:** 2

Panzanella is usually a no-fuss mix of cucumbers, onions, tomatoes, and bread. Here, I take the bread salad idea and amp it up with loads of superfoods and a sweet and tangy berry dressing.

For the dressing

½ cup fresh blueberries

¼ cup balsamic vinegar

1 tablespoon chia seeds

⅛ teaspoon freshly
 ground black pepper

Pinch salt

1 teaspoon pure
 maple syrup

For the salad

2 whole-grain bread slices

1½ cup greens, such as
 baby spinach

½ cup chickpeas, drained
 and rinsed

¼ cup broccoli florets

¼ cup cauliflower florets

2 tablespoons
 shredded cabbage

2 tablespoons sliced
 grape tomatoes

2 tablespoons
 pumpkin seeds

2 tablespoons
 broccoli sprouts

2 tablespoons sliced
 onion, rinsed

1 cup cooked quinoa
 (page 137)

1. **Make the dressing:** In a blender, combine the blueberries, vinegar, chia seeds, pepper, salt, and maple syrup and blend until smooth. Set aside.

2. **Make the salad:** Place the bread in a cold oven, and preheat to 350°F. Once the oven has reached the temperature, flip the bread over and toast for an additional 5 minutes.

3. Meanwhile, evenly divide the greens, chickpeas, broccoli, cauliflower, cabbage, tomatoes, pumpkin seeds, broccoli sprouts, and onion between two plates. Add ½ cup of cooked quinoa (warm or cold) to each plate.

4. Remove the bread from the oven and cut into cubes. Top each salad with the bread and half of the blueberry dressing. Serve.

PREPARATION TIP: Rinsing cut onions gives them a subtler flavor and can help ease digestion.

PER SERVING: Calories: 411; Total fat: 10g; Total carbs: 65g; Fiber: 13g; Sugar: 16g; Protein: 17g; Sodium: 333mg

Southwest-Inspired Spinach Salad

PREP TIME: 10 minutes **SERVES:** 2

Sweet and smoky, this salad does not disappoint. Brown rice and black beans make this a filling, satisfying dinner. Flaxseed adds a nice crunch and some omega-3 and omega-6 fatty acids, which help with cardiovascular ailments, such a lowering blood pressure and bad cholesterol. They are small but mighty!

½ tablespoon balsamic vinegar

½ tablespoon Barbecue Sauce (page 19)

½ teaspoon smoked paprika

¼ teaspoon red pepper flakes

8 ounces fresh spinach

½ cup black beans, drained and rinsed

½ cup cooked brown rice (page 137)

½ cup sweet corn

½ tablespoon whole flaxseed or sesame seeds

1. In a large bowl, whisk together the vinegar, barbecue sauce, paprika, and red pepper flakes. Mix in the spinach, beans, rice, and corn. Toss well to coat.

2. Top with the flaxseed and serve.

SHORTCUT: Use a store-bought oil-free barbecue sauce in place of the homemade version in a pinch.

VARIATION TIP: Pinto beans would make an excellent substitute for the black beans. If you like onions, a few sliced red onions also add a nice crunch to the salad.

PER SERVING: Calories: 313; Total fat: 4g; Total carbs: 61g; Fiber: 9g; Sugar: 4g; Protein: 12g; Sodium: 143mg

Lentil and Potato Hash

30 MINUTES **GLUTEN-FREE** **NUT-FREE** **ONE POT** **SOY-FREE**

PREP TIME: 10 minutes **COOK TIME:** 15 minutes **SERVES:** 4

Starchy potatoes and tender brown lentils come together for a surprisingly easy meal that really stands out from the crowd. Russet potatoes tend to hold their shape better, but a sweet potato would add a delicious twist—simply decrease your potato cooking time, so the sweet potato doesn't get too mushy.

¼ cup vegetable broth or water, plus more as needed

1 (10-ounce) russet potato, unpeeled and cut into ¼-inch pieces

1 teaspoon ground cumin

½ teaspoon ground allspice

½ teaspoon ground ginger

½ teaspoon garam masala

½ teaspoon salt or Salt-Free Spice Blend (page 14)

1 (15-ounce) can brown lentils, drained and rinsed

½ cup chopped scallions, green and white parts

½ cup chopped fresh cilantro (optional)

¼ cup chopped unsalted peanuts (optional)

1. In a large skillet, heat the broth over medium-high heat. Add the potato, cumin, allspice, ginger, garam masala, and salt. Cook, stirring frequently, for about 10 minutes, until the potato is tender. Add more broth or water as needed to maintain a very thick sauce consistency.

2. Add the lentils and stir to combine. Lower the heat to medium, cover, and cook for 5 minutes more.

3. Divide the lentil mixture among four bowls. Top each serving with 2 tablespoons of scallions, 2 tablespoons of cilantro (if using), and 1 tablespoon of peanuts (if using), then serve.

SHORTCUT: Use a store-bought salt-free spice blend in place of the homemade version in a pinch.

VARIATION TIP: You can do a lot of fun things with this recipe. If you love mung beans (I do!), use 1½ cups cooked mung beans to replace the lentils. Or to go for an entirely different flavor profile, use pinto beans and replace the allspice, ginger, and garam masala with ½ teaspoon each of ground cinnamon, chipotle chile powder, and chili powder.

PER SERVING: Calories: 148; Total fat: 1g; Total carbs: 29g; Fiber: 7g; Sugar: 2g; Protein: 8g; Sodium: 28mg

One-Pot Shakshuka

30 MINUTES GLUTEN-FREE NUT-FREE ONE POT SOY-FREE

PREP TIME: 10 minutes **COOK TIME:** 20 minutes **SERVES:** 6

Shakshuka is traditionally a dish of poached eggs cooked in a spiced tomato sauce. Here I create a zesty tomato sauce and use chickpeas for the protein.

1 onion, diced

3 garlic cloves, finely chopped

1 green bell pepper, diced

1 jalapeño pepper, seeded and diced

2 bay leaves

2 to 3 tablespoons tomato paste

1½ tablespoons paprika

1 tablespoon ground cumin

1 teaspoon chili powder

1 teaspoon freshly ground black pepper

1 (28-ounce) can crushed tomatoes

2 tablespoons finely chopped fresh cilantro

1 (15-ounce) can chickpeas, drained and rinsed

¼ to ½ cup kalamata or green olives, coarsely chopped (optional)

1. In a large skillet over medium-high heat, combine the onion, garlic, bell pepper, and jalapeño and cook, stirring, for about 3 minutes, until the onion is soft but not browned. Add 1 to 2 tablespoons of water as needed to prevent burning. Add the bay leaves and sauté for 30 seconds.

2. Add 2 tablespoons of tomato paste. Cook for 2 minutes, stirring constantly. If you want a thicker sauce, add 1 more tablespoon of tomato paste.

3. Stir in the paprika, cumin, chili powder, and black pepper and cook for 1 minute. Carefully pour in the tomatoes with their juices. Cover the skillet and turn the heat to low. Cook for 10 minutes, stirring occasionally.

4. Remove from the heat and discard the bay leaves. Stir in the cilantro, chickpeas, and olives (if using). Serve warm.

PREPARATION TIP: This sauce is thick and tends to splatter, so you'll benefit from using a lid and splatter guard in the final steps. Having all ingredients prepped also helps you avoid scorching the onions and garlic and splattering the thick sauce as it simmers.

PER SERVING: Calories: 130; Total fat: 2g; Total carbs: 25g; Fiber: 7g; Sugar: 7g; Protein: 7g; Sodium: 254mg

Four-Can Chili

EASY PREP **FREEZES WELL** **GLUTEN-FREE** **NUT-FREE** **ONE POT** **SOY-FREE**

PREP TIME: 5 minutes **COOK TIME:** 30 minutes **SERVES:** 6

It doesn't get much easier than this: four cans, some spices, and a large pot. I love to make chili and then use it in different ways throughout the week. One night I might enjoy a simple bowl of chili, and then the next night, I might use it to top a baked potato or bowl of brown rice. Variety is the spice of plant-based diets!

1 (28-ounce) can crushed
tomatoes

1 (15-ounce) can
black beans

1 (15-ounce) can
cannellini beans

1 (15-ounce) can
chickpeas

1 tablespoon chili powder

1 teaspoon garlic powder

1 teaspoon onion powder

½ teaspoon
ground cumin

½ teaspoon red pepper
flakes (optional)

In a large stockpot, combine the tomatoes, black beans, cannellini beans, and chickpeas and their liquids. Add the chili powder, garlic powder, onion powder, cumin, and red pepper flakes (if using). Bring the chili to a boil over medium-high heat. Cover, reduce the heat to medium-low, and simmer for 25 minutes, until the flavors meld. Serve.

INGREDIENT TIP: To use dried beans instead of canned, soak ½ cup each of dried black beans, dried cannellini beans, and dried chickpeas overnight, then drain, rinse, and put them in the pot with 5 cups of vegetable broth or water, the spices, and the tomatoes. After the chili comes to a boil, reduce the heat and simmer for 45 to 60 minutes, or until the beans are tender while still holding their form.

PER SERVING: Calories: 216; Total fat: 2g; Total carbs: 39g; Fiber: 15g; Sugar: 6g; Protein: 13g; Sodium: 195mg

Tex-Mex Quinoa Vegetable Soup

FREEZES WELL GLUTEN-FREE NUT-FREE ONE POT SOY-FREE

PREP TIME: 20 minutes **COOK TIME:** 6 to 8 hours in a slow cooker **SERVES:** 6

Warm and comforting, this soup is exactly what you want on a chilly day. You can make it ahead in your slow cooker or cook it on the stove-top (see tip). Both variations are absolute crowd-pleasers. Quinoa is considered a protein-heavy "grain," but—fun fact—it is technically a protein-heavy seed!

1 cup quinoa

½ large onion, diced

2 garlic cloves, minced

2 carrots, cut into coins

2 celery stalks, sliced

1 tablespoon water, plus more as needed

¼ cup tomato paste

1 zucchini, cut into coins and quartered

1 (14-ounce) can whole-kernel corn, drained

1 (14-ounce) can diced tomatoes

1 (15-ounce) can black beans, drained and rinsed

1 (15-ounce) can red kidney beans, drained and rinsed

2 teaspoons chili powder

1 teaspoon ground cumin

6 cups vegetable broth, plus more as needed

1. Place the quinoa in a fine-mesh sieve and rinse under cold water for 2 to 3 minutes, or until the cloudy water becomes clear.

2. On a 5-quart or larger slow cooker, set the temperature to High and let it heat for 5 to 10 minutes.

3. In the preheated slow cooker, combine the onion, garlic, carrots, celery, and water and cook for 2 to 3 minutes. Stir in the tomato paste to combine.

4. Add the rinsed quinoa, zucchini, corn, tomatoes, black beans, kidney beans, chili powder, cumin, and broth. Stir well. The tomato paste will fully incorporate as the soup cooks.

5. Set the heat to Low. Cover the slow cooker and cook on Low for 6 to 8 hours (or on High for 3 to 4 hours). If the soup seems too thick, add more broth or water, ½ cup at a time. Serve warm.

INGREDIENT TIP: Black beans and kidney beans are the most common types used for Tex-Mex–style meals, but use any variety you like. Give this recipe a kick with jalapeño peppers or other hot peppers.

PREPARATION TIP: To cook this soup on the stovetop, follow steps 1 through 5, but in step 5, cook the soup over medium-low heat, covered, for 45 to 60 minutes. Stir occasionally to prevent the tomatoes from settling to the bottom and scorching.

PER SERVING: Calories: 299; Total fat: 3g; Total carbs: 56g; Fiber: 14g; Sugar: 7g; Protein: 15g; Sodium: 230mg

Quinoa Pilaf

30 MINUTES **GLUTEN-FREE** **ONE POT** **SOY-FREE**

PREP TIME: 10 minutes **COOK TIME:** 20 minutes **SERVES:** 4

Inspired by traditional pilaf dishes of rice or wheat, this vegetable-packed quinoa is the answer to the weeknight "What's for dinner?" question. The walnuts' crunch is texturally pleasing, and they are also high in antioxidants and are a great source of omega-3 fatty acids. Truth be told, I love the addition of fresh herbs as a garnish for flavor, and also because they make the dish seem fancy.

½ cup chopped red onion

1 cup diced carrots

½ teaspoon dried parsley

½ teaspoon dried thyme

1 cup dry quinoa, rinsed
    and drained

1½ cups vegetable broth

¼ cup chopped walnuts

Chopped fresh parsley or
    thyme, for garnish

1. In a large saucepan over medium-high heat, add the onion and carrots and cook, stirring frequently, for 3 to 5 minutes until softened. Add 1 to 2 tablespoons of water as needed to prevent burning. Add the parsley, thyme, quinoa, and broth and bring to a boil.

2. Reduce the heat to medium-low, cover, and cook for 15 minutes.

3. Remove the pan from the heat and let sit for 5 minutes.

4. Fluff the quinoa with a fork, then add the walnuts and gently mix until combined.

5. Spoon into bowls and serve garnished with fresh parsley.

VARIATION TIP: If you like to cook plain grains in bulk— think rice, farro, and millet—you can transform them by sautéing onion and carrot in a skillet as directed here, adding 1 or 2 cups cooked grains (no vegetable broth), and stir-frying until hot.

PER SERVING: Calories: 226; Total fat: 7g; Total carbs: 33g; Fiber: 5g; Sugar: 3g; Protein: 8g; Sodium: 40mg

Easy Mushroom Farro-tto

NUT-FREE ONE POT SOY-FREE

PREP TIME: 10 minutes **COOK TIME:** 45 minutes **SERVES:** 4

Traditional risotto dishes use arborio white rice and a constant stirring method to release the starch, which yields a creamy texture. Using farro and letting it cook covered releases its starch and then adding nutritional yeast produces a creaminess without stirring—what a win! The combination of mushrooms and shallots gives this dish a rich, savory flavor, and the rosemary adds a brightness that complements the umami-rich mushrooms.

8 ounces cremini mush-
  rooms, sliced

1 shallot, thinly sliced
  (about ¼ cup)

2 sprigs rosemary,
  chopped (about
  1 tablespoon)

¼ cup water

2 cups vegetable broth

1 cup pearled farro

2 tablespoons nutritional
  yeast

1. In a saucepan or Dutch oven over medium-high heat, combine the mushrooms, shallot, rosemary, and water and cook, stirring frequently, for about 5 minutes, until the mushrooms are glistening.

2. Add the broth and farro and bring to a boil. Reduce the heat to low, cover, and simmer for 30 minutes, until the farro is tender.

3. Add the nutritional yeast and simmer, uncovered, for 5 to 7 minutes, until most of the liquid evaporates and you have a creamy grain dish. Serve warm.

PER SERVING: Calories: 190; Total fat: 1g; Total carbs: 41g; Fiber: 8g; Sugar: 2g; Protein: 8g; Sodium: 33mg

Mango-Ginger Chickpea Curry

30 MINUTES EASY PREP GLUTEN-FREE NUT-FREE ONE POT SOY-FREE

PREP TIME: 5 minutes **COOK TIME:** 15 minutes **SERVES:** 6

Sweet mango and spicy ginger are brought together in this tasty curry dish. I love to serve it over nutty brown rice. Using plant-based milk versus full-fat or lite coconut milk (as traditional curries use) keeps the fat content down, but maintains all the flavor.

2 (15-ounce) cans
chickpeas, drained
and rinsed

2 cups fresh or frozen
mango chunks

2 cups unsweetened
plant-based milk

2 tablespoons pure
maple syrup

1 tablespoon
curry powder

1 tablespoon
ground ginger

1 teaspoon ground
coriander

1 teaspoon garlic powder

1 teaspoon onion powder

⅛ teaspoon ground
cinnamon

1. In a large stock pot or Dutch oven over medium heat, combine the chickpeas, mango, milk, maple syrup, curry powder, ginger, coriander, garlic powder, onion powder, and cinnamon. Cover and cook for 10 minutes, stirring after about 5 minutes.

2. Uncover and cook for an additional 5 minutes, stirring every other minute, until the flavors meld. Serve.

PREPARATION TIP: You can cook this curry in an electric pressure cooker on Manual for 30 minutes. It can also be prepared in a slow cooker and cooked on High for 4 to 6 hours.

PER SERVING: Calories: 201; Total fat: 4g; Total carbs: 35g; Fiber: 7g; Sugar: 17g; Protein: 8g; Sodium: 204mg

One-Pot Spaghetti Dinner

30 MINUTES EASY PREP NUT-FREE ONE POT SOY-FREE

PREP TIME: 5 minutes **COOK TIME:** 20 minutes **SERVES:** 4

Colander-free, one-pot spaghetti is my go-to dinner. Living in a tiny home without a dishwasher, I had to figure out how to make spaghetti—my favorite dish!—without dirtying a pot for sauce, a pot for spaghetti, and a colander. Using this recipe's ratio of water and tomatoes led to an impeccably saucy spaghetti. I like my spaghetti tender, so when I use boxed spaghetti, I typically cook it for about 5 minutes over the cooking time. If you prefer yours al dente, reduce cooking time by 2 minutes and reduce the water by ¼ cup.

2 (15-ounce) cans crushed tomatoes

4 cups water

1 (15-ounce) can great northern beans, drained but not rinsed

1 (16-ounce) box whole-grain spaghetti pasta

3 tablespoons dried basil

2 garlic cloves, minced

1 tablespoon nutritional yeast

1 teaspoon onion powder

⅛ teaspoon salt

1. In a shallow 10- to 12-inch sauté pan or skillet, combine the tomatoes, water, beans, spaghetti, basil, garlic, nutritional yeast, onion powder, and salt.

2. Bring to a boil over high heat, then reduce the heat to medium. Simmer for 16 to 19 minutes, until the pasta is tender and the sauce has thickened.

3. Remove from heat and serve warm.

INGREDIENT TIP: Prefer to use your favorite pasta sauce? Substitute a 24-ounce jar of store-bought oil-free pasta sauce, plus ¾ cup of water for the tomatoes, basil, garlic, and onion powder.

PER SERVING: Calories: 576; Total fat: 3g; Total carbs: 116g; Fiber: 13g; Sugar: 13g; Protein: 24g; Sodium: 508mg

Chickpea al Pastor Tacos

GLUTEN-FREE NUT-FREE ONE POT SOY-FREE

PREP TIME: 10 minutes **COOK TIME:** 30 minutes **SERVES:** 4

Al pastor is traditionally a rotisserie-style meat-based dish with onions and pineapples. Here I use roasted chickpeas as a plant-based replacement. Adding the pineapple and onion to the baking sheet yields caramelized and slightly charred accompaniments to the chickpeas. Adding the seasonings part-way through the cooking process keeps them from burning while still giving them time to infuse.

2 (15-ounce) cans chickpeas, drained and rinsed

½ red onion, sliced

1 (15-ounce) can crushed pineapple, drained and divided

2 tablespoons liquid aminos

½ teaspoon ground cumin

¼ teaspoon garlic powder

¼ teaspoon dried oregano

¼ teaspoon freshly ground black pepper

⅛ teaspoon ground cinnamon

Pinch of ground cloves

12 oil-free corn tortillas, wrapped in parchment paper

¼ to ⅓ cup pineapple or mango salsa

1. Preheat the oven to 400°F and line a baking sheet with parchment paper.

2. Spread the chickpeas, onion, and pineapple on the prepared baking sheet.

3. Bake for 15 to 20 minutes, until the chickpeas start to break open.

4. Drizzle the liquid aminos over the chickpeas, pineapple, and onions. Evenly sprinkle the cumin, garlic powder, oregano, pepper, cinnamon, and cloves over all, then stir carefully with a rubber spatula to incorporate. Place the wrapped tortillas on top of the chickpea mixture, and bake for 5 to 7 minutes, until the chickpeas and pineapple have started to brown slightly.

5. Scoop the chickpea, pineapple, and onion mixture into the tortillas and serve with the salsa.

INGREDIENT TIP: Make your own fresh pineapple salsa: In a small bowl, mix together ¼ cup of rinsed finely diced red onion, ¼ cup of chopped fresh pineapple, 2 tablespoons of chopped fresh cilantro, 1 teaspoon of pineapple juice, and 1 teaspoon of lime juice.

PER SERVING: Calories: 377; Total fat: 5g; Total carbs: 74g; Fiber: 12g; Sugar: 16g; Protein: 13g; Sodium: 252mg

Sheet Pan Fajitas

EASY PREP **GLUTEN-FREE** **NUT-FREE** **ONE POT** **SOY-FREE**

PREP TIME: 5 minutes **COOK TIME:** 30 minutes **SERVES:** 2

Fajitas have always been a favorite of mine—who can resist those fragrant, sizzling cast-iron platters of veggies? Here, I take my favorite fillings—mushrooms, bell pepper, and onion—and roast them to caramelized perfection, toss them in a tasty seasoning, and pair them with crunchy cabbage and creamy avocado for the ideal meal.

8 ounces portabella
   mushrooms, sliced

1 red bell pepper, sliced

½ red onion, sliced

6 oil-free corn tortillas

2 tablespoons
   liquid aminos

1 tablespoon freshly
   squeezed lime juice

1 teaspoon ground cumin

1 cup shredded cabbage

1 avocado, pitted, peeled,
   and sliced

Lime wedges, for serving

1. Preheat the oven to 400°F and line a baking sheet with parchment paper.

2. Spread the mushrooms, pepper, and onion evenly on the prepared baking sheet in a single layer.

3. Bake for 20 to 25 minutes, until the mushrooms are glistening and the peppers and onions are tender and starting to brown.

4. Wrap the tortillas in parchment paper and place them on top of the vegetables. Bake for an additional 5 minutes.

5. Remove the wrapped tortillas. Drizzle the liquid aminos and lime juice on top of the vegetables, then sprinkle with cumin. Stir and serve scooped into tortillas and topped with cabbage, avocado, and lime wedges.

VARIATION TIP: You could certainly add other vegetables, or even drained and rinsed beans, to enhance these flavorful fajitas.

PER SERVING: Calories: 398; Total fat: 18g; Total carbs: 57g; Fiber: 15g; Sugar: 9g; Protein: 10g; Sodium: 42mg

Stuffed Sweet Potatoes

GLUTEN-FREE NUT-FREE ONE POT SOY-FREE

PREP TIME: 10 minutes **COOK TIME:** 45 minutes **SERVES:** 4

This sheet pan meal is a tried-and-true dinner in my house. I love to make a double batch and eat it throughout the week as my quick-prepped lunch or easy-reheat dinner. This meal can satisfy two hungry people or four people when accompanied by a dinner salad or Lemony Kale Salad (page 31).

2 sweet potatoes (roughly 2 inches in diameter)

¼ teaspoon freshly ground black pepper, divided

1 (15-ounce) can black beans, drained and rinsed

1 ½ cups cauliflower florets

1 ½ cups broccoli florets

¼ cup chopped onion

¼ teaspoon salt

½ batch Go-To Bowl Sauce (page 16)

1. Preheat the oven to 400° F and line a baking sheet with parchment paper.

2. Halve the sweet potatoes lengthwise and season with ⅛ teaspoon of pepper, then place them cut-side down and evenly spaced on the baking sheet. Poke the skin with a fork.

3. Bake for 15 minutes. Add the beans, cauliflower, broccoli, and onion to the baking sheet in a single layer. Season with the salt and remaining ⅛ teaspoon of pepper.

4. Bake for 20 to 30 minutes, until the potatoes are soft and a knife slides in easily. The vegetables will begin to brown and the beans should start to crack.

5. Serve the potatoes, cut-side up, with the vegetables and beans layered on top. Drizzle with 2 tablespoons of Go-To Bowl Sauce and enjoy.

SHORTCUT: Don't have time to make the bowl sauce? A simple drizzle of tahini will do the trick!

PER SERVING: Calories: 167; Total fat: 2g; Total carbs: 34g; Fiber: 10g; Sugar: 5g; Protein: 9g; Sodium: 206mg

Barbecue Sweet Potato Bowl

5 INGREDIENT **GLUTEN-FREE** **NUT-FREE** **ONE POT** **SOY-FREE**

PREP TIME: 10 minutes **COOK TIME:** 30 minutes **SERVES:** 4

Rich barbecue sauce complements the roasted sweet potatoes, broccoli, and chickpeas in this super-easy dinner bowl. Roasting all the ingredients at once yields tender sweet potatoes, crispy broccoli, and hearty chickpeas. I load them all in a bowl and drizzle them with barbecue sauce for a dinner that is ready in about 30 minutes.

3 pounds sweet potatoes, peeled and cubed

2 cups broccoli florets

1 (15-ounce) can chickpeas, drained and rinsed

1 cup Barbecue Sauce (page 19), warmed

1. Preheat the oven to 400°F and line a baking sheet with parchment paper.

2. Arrange the potatoes, broccoli, and chickpeas into a single layer on the prepared baking sheet.

3. Bake for 30 minutes, or until the sweet potatoes are knife-tender.

4. Plate the vegetables and drizzle ¼ cup of barbecue sauce on each serving. Serve.

PREPARATION TIP: Use precut broccoli florets, often found in your produce section, to make this dinner even quicker.

SHORTCUT: Use an oil-free store-bought barbecue sauce in place of the homemade version.

PER SERVING: Calories: 448; Total fat: 2g; Total carbs: 99g; Fiber: 16g; Sugar: 10g; Protein: 11g; Sodium: 323mg

Roasted Kabocha Squash with Chickpeas

5 INGREDIENT GLUTEN-FREE NUT-FREE ONE POT SOY-FREE

PREP TIME: 10 minutes **COOK TIME:** 40 minutes **SERVES:** 4

Aquafaba, or chickpea liquid, is a plant-based miracle. It can be found in recipes for everything from baking to salad dressings, but I use it here to help the squash retain its moisture while roasting and to help the seasonings stick. To collect aquafaba, simply strain off the liquid from your chickpeas, reserve, and use as needed.

2 (15-ounce) cans chickpeas

1 (2- to 3-pound) kabocha squash

½ teaspoon salt

¼ teaspoon freshly ground black pepper

2 teaspoons smoked paprika

2 teaspoons garlic powder

1. Preheat the oven to 400°F. Line a baking sheet with parchment paper.

2. Open both cans of chickpeas and drain, reserving 2 tablespoons of the aquafaba. Transfer the chickpeas to a zip-top bag.

3. Wash the squash very well. Cut it in half. Remove the seeds with a spoon and discard. Remove the stem, then slice each half lengthwise to create 1-inch-thick wedges. Place the wedges on the prepared baking sheet. Drizzle with 1 tablespoon of the aquafaba. Toss with tongs to coat all sides. Sprinkle with salt and pepper. Bake for 20 minutes.

4. While the squash bakes, add the remaining 1 tablespoon of aquafaba, the paprika, and garlic powder to the bag with the chickpeas. Close and shake gently, until the chickpeas are coated.

5. Remove the baking sheet from the oven. Flip the squash over and pour the chickpeas onto the baking sheet, spreading them into a single layer around the squash. Bake for 15 to 20 minutes, until the chickpeas are just beginning to brown and the squash is tender. Serve warm.

VARIATION TIP: Play with flavor profiles. Try a combination of ground ginger and shichimi togarashi (also sold as Japanese 7-spice blend) or a mixture of curry powder, turmeric, and garam masala. Just make sure you use 4 teaspoons of spices total.

PER SERVING: Calories: 256; Total fat: 3g; Total carbs: 51g; Fiber: 11g; Sugar: 5g; Protein: 10g; Sodium: 398mg

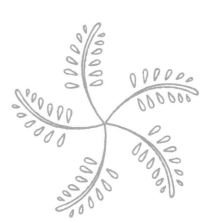

Greek-Inspired Roasted Potatoes and Vegetables

EASY PREP **GLUTEN-FREE** **NUT-FREE** **ONE POT** **SOY-FREE**

PREP TIME: 10 minutes **COOK TIME:** 30 minutes **SERVES:** 4

Lemony potatoes with savory oregano whisk you away to Mykonos or Crete. Inspired by the flavors of the Mediterranean—lemon, olives, and artichokes—this potato dish is vibrant in both flavor and color.

1 pound yellow potatoes, cut into 1-inch cubes

½ cup diced red bell pepper

1 (15.5-ounce) can quartered artichokes, drained

1 (15-ounce) can chickpeas, drained and rinsed

1 (4-ounce) can sliced black olives

½ cup sliced red onion

2 garlic cloves, minced

¼ cup freshly squeezed lemon juice

1 cup vegetable broth

1 teaspoon dried oregano

1. Preheat the oven to 400°F.

2. In a roasting pan, stir together the potatoes, bell pepper, artichokes, chickpeas, olives, onion, and garlic. Drizzle the lemon juice and broth on top, then sprinkle on the oregano. Stir to combine.

3. Bake for 20 to 30 minutes, until the potatoes are knife-tender and the liquids are mostly evaporated. Serve warm.

VARIATION TIP: You can add fresh vegetables, such as green beans or summer squash, to up the vegetable quantity in this dish.

PER SERVING: Calories: 265; Total fat: 5g; Total carbs: 50g; Fiber: 16g; Sugar: 6g; Protein: 10g; Sodium: 393mg

Shake and Bake Tofu Dinner

5 INGREDIENT **NUT-FREE** **ONE POT**

PREP TIME: 10 minutes **COOK TIME:** 40 minutes **SERVES:** 4

Let's take it back to pure ease and convenience: remember those Shake 'n Bake seasoning boxes? This recipe is inspired by that nostalgic dinner favorite, using tofu, potatoes, and green beans to evoke classic comfort food. I love the combination of crispy panko bread crumbs with soft tofu. With all the textures and flavors of the original, you won't miss the meat!

1 cup panko bread crumbs

1 tablespoon nutritional yeast

1 tablespoon Salt-Free Spice Blend (page 14)

1 (14-ounce) block firm tofu, drained

1 pound potatoes, cut into ½-inch cubes

1 pound fresh green beans, trimmed

1. Preheat the oven to 400°F and line a baking sheet with parchment paper.

2. In a zip-top bag, mix together the bread crumbs, nutritional yeast, and salt-free spice blend.

3. Cut the tofu into eight equal slabs, then toss in the bread crumb mixture until evenly coated.

4. Carefully place the tofu on one side of the prepared baking sheet in a single layer. Add the potatoes to the other side.

5. Bake for 20 minutes, remove from the oven, and carefully flip the tofu over. Add the green beans and bake an additional 15 to 20 minutes, until the tofu starts to brown and the potatoes are knife-tender. Serve warm.

VARIATION TIP: Any fresh vegetables will work in this recipe. Simply adjust the time at which you add them to the baking sheet to ensure they roast to their ideal texture.

PER SERVING: Calories: 257; Total fat: 5g; Total carbs: 41g; Fiber: 7g; Sugar: 6g; Protein: 15g; Sodium: 144mg

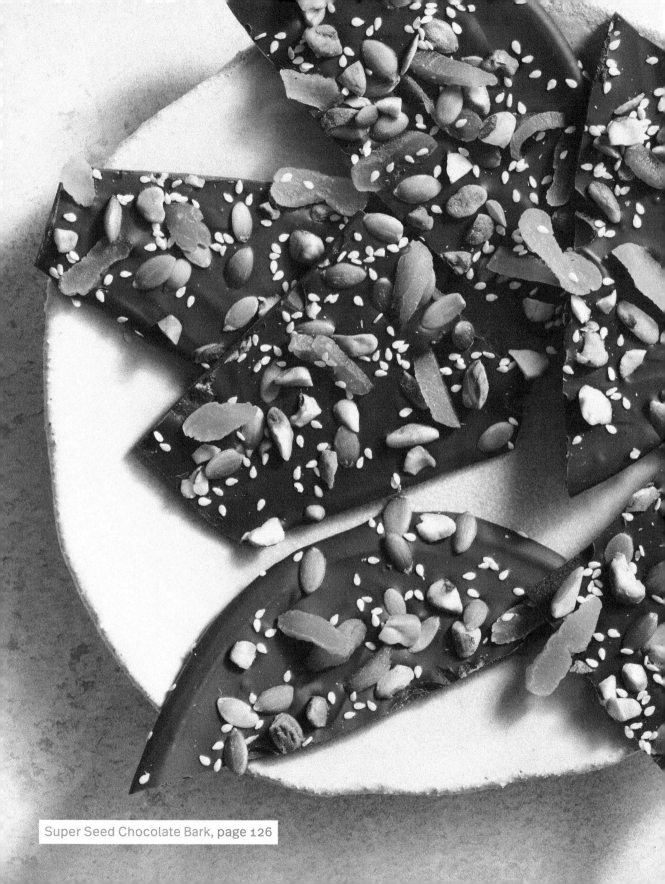

Super Seed Chocolate Bark, page 126

CHAPTER 7

Super Easy Snacks and Desserts

Kale Chips

5 INGREDIENT **30 MINUTES** **EASY PREP** **GLUTEN-FREE** **NUT-FREE** **SOY-FREE**

PREP TIME: 5 minutes **COOK TIME:** 20 minutes **SERVES:** 4

Crunchy, savory kale chips are always a fun snack. These come together quickly and taste delicious. You can eat them on their own or use them as a crunchy salad topper. Kale is high in antioxidants and vitamins and retains its nutritional value when baked. These oil-free snacks are an excellent way to eat your greens!

¼ cup vegetable broth

1 tablespoon nutritional yeast

½ teaspoon garlic powder

½ teaspoon onion powder

6 ounces kale, stemmed and cut into 2- to 3-inch pieces

1. Preheat the oven to 300°F. Line a baking sheet with parchment paper.

2. In a small bowl, mix together the broth, nutritional yeast, garlic powder, and onion powder.

3. Put the kale in a large bowl. Pour the broth and seasonings over the kale, and toss well to thoroughly coat.

4. Place the kale pieces on the prepared baking sheet in an even layer. Bake, turning the kale halfway through, for 20 minutes, or until crispy. Serve.

VARIATION TIP: For a smoky flavor, add 1 teaspoon of smoked paprika to the recipe. To create spicy kale chips, add ½ teaspoon of red pepper flakes.

PER SERVING: Calories: 34; Total fat: 0g; Total carbs: 6g; Fiber: 2g; Sugar: 1g; Protein: 2g; Sodium: 75mg

Beet Chips

PREP TIME: 15 minutes **COOK TIME:** 15 minutes **SERVES:** 4

Crispy beet chips are perfect for snacking and dipping. Using aquafaba (the liquid from a can of chickpeas) helps the herbs and spices stick to the beets, making this an oil-free snack you'll make again and again. You can use the leftover chickpeas to whip up a batch of the White Bean and Chickpea Hummus (page 124) to pair with your beet chips.

4 medium beets, scrubbed

3 tablespoons aquafaba

1 teaspoon dried dill

1 teaspoon dried chives

1 teaspoon dried parsley

1 teaspoon cayenne pepper

1. Preheat the oven to 375°F. Line two baking sheets with parchment paper.

2. Using a mandoline or sharp knife, cut the beets into $\frac{1}{16}$-inch-thick slices. Transfer to a large bowl.

3. Add the aquafaba, dill, chives, parsley, and cayenne pepper, and toss until evenly coated.

4. Arrange the beet slices in a single layer on the prepared baking sheets. Bake for 15 minutes, until they begin to curl and crisp. Serve.

SHORTCUT: Air fryer fans, this one's for you! Preheat your air fryer to 400° F. Transfer the beet slices to an unlined air fryer basket and cook for 8 minutes, shaking every 2 minutes, until crispy.

PER SERVING: Calories: 44; Total fat: 0g; Total carbs: 9g; Fiber: 3g; Sugar: 6g; Protein: 2g; Sodium: 65mg

Savory Snack Mix

EASY PREP **SOY-FREE**

MAKES ABOUT 5 CUPS **PREP TIME:** 5 minutes **COOK TIME:** 1 hour

I love a savory, crunchy snack, but so many of them are packed with oil and butter. Pairing tahini with umami-rich vegan Worcestershire sauce and spices yields a zesty snack mix. I was able to find puffed "O" vegan cereal without added sugar in several grocery stores to use for the puffed cereal in this mix. I use a whole-grain wheat bran cereal for the second cereal, which offsets the puffed cereal with its flat and super crunchy texture. Mix and match the cereals you can find for your perfect go-to snack mix.

2 cups puffed
  vegan cereal
1 cup whole-grain
  crunchy cereal
1 cup raw unsalted nuts
½ cup oil-free pretzels
½ cup pumpkin seeds
1 tablespoon tahini
1 tablespoon water
1 tablespoon vegan
  Worcestershire sauce
1 tablespoon Salt-Free
  Spice Blend (page 14)
¼ teaspoon garlic powder
¼ teaspoon onion powder

1. Preheat the oven to 275°F.

2. In a baking dish or roasting pan, mix together the puffed cereal, crunchy cereal, nuts, pretzels, and seeds.

3. In a small bowl, whisk together the tahini, water, and Worcestershire sauce.

4. Pour the tahini mixture over the cereal mixture and toss to coat. Sprinkle the salt-free spice blend, garlic powder, and onion powder over the cereal mixture and stir to combine.

5. Bake for 1 hour, stirring every 15 minutes, until the cereal mixture is crispy.

6. Allow the snack mix to cool completely in the pan, then serve.

SHORTCUT: Use a store-bought salt-free spice blend plus 1 teaspoon of nutritional yeast in place of the homemade version.

VARIATION TIP: I mix up my nuts when I make this. Sometimes I use all cashews, and other times I use ¼ cup each of four different nuts (cashews, walnuts, pistachios, and pecans). Sliced almonds also work really well. If you can't find a vegan Worcestershire, Pickapeppa hot sauce is a great substitute.

PER SERVING (½ CUP): Calories: 165; Total fat: 11g; Total carbs: 14g; Fiber: 2g; Sugar: 1g; Protein: 6g; Sodium: 47mg

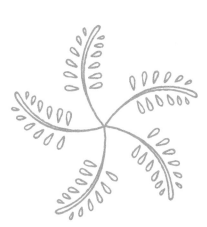

Lonestar Bean Dip

30 MINUTES **GLUTEN-FREE** **NO COOK** **NUT-FREE** **ONE POT** **SOY-FREE**

PREP TIME: 10 minutes **SERVES:** 4

I tend to steer clear of conventional bean dips coated with oily dressings and instead bring this version to parties and potlucks. It also makes a great grab-and-go snack right out of the refrigerator. This bean dip is bound to be a favorite, from the crunchy celery to the tangy seasoned rice vinegar. I like to pair it with large ribs of celery or hearty crackers for scooping.

1 (15-ounce can) black-eyed peas, drained and rinsed

½ cup finely chopped celery

½ cup sweet corn

¼ cup packed finely chopped massaged kale

¼ cup finely chopped bell pepper (any color)

¼ cup finely chopped red onion

1 (4-ounce) pimentos, drained and chopped

1 garlic clove, minced

3 tablespoons seasoned rice vinegar

½ teaspoon Salt-Free Spice Blend (page 14)

½ teaspoon chili powder

Celery sticks, crackers, or baked tostadas, for serving

1. In a medium bowl, mix the black-eye peas, celery, corn, kale, bell pepper, onion, pimentos, and garlic until well combined.

2. Stir in the vinegar, salt-free spice blend, and chili powder.

3. Serve with celery.

SHORTCUT: Use a store-bought salt-free spice blend in place of the homemade version.

PER SERVING: Calories: 121; Total fat: 1g; Total carbs: 23g; Fiber: 8g; Sugar: 3g; Protein: 7g; Sodium: 30mg

Baba Ghanoush

5 INGREDIENT **GLUTEN-FREE** **NUT-FREE** **SOY-FREE**

PREP TIME: 10 minutes **COOK TIME:** 1 hour 5 minutes **SERVES:** 4

I enjoy creamy dips, but I don't always love to get out my blender or food processor to make them. By baking an eggplant until the inside is creamy, you can mash it with a fork to yield a creamy roasted dip. Traditional baba ghanoush is made with oil, but I've found with the right amount of tahini and lemon juice, I can achieve a delightful dip without it. Pair this with cut veggies, crackers, or whole-grain pitas.

1 (1-pound) eggplant
2 tablespoons tahini
1 tablespoon freshly
  squeezed lemon juice
1 teaspoon ground cumin
½ teaspoon dried parsley

1. Preheat the oven to 400°F and line a baking sheet with parchment paper.

2. With a fork, pierce the eggplant's skin a few times on each side and place it on the prepared baking sheet. Roast for 60 to 75 minutes, until the inside of the eggplant is soft and gooey, and the outside has started to brown and is crispy. The gooier the inside, the easier it will be to mash.

3. Remove the eggplant from the oven and carefully remove the skin.

4. In a medium bowl, mash the eggplant with a fork, separating any fibrous sections.

5. Stir in the tahini, lemon juice, cumin, and parsley, then serve.

PER SERVING: Calories: 76; Total fat: 5g; Total carbs: 9g; Fiber: 4g; Sugar: 4g; Protein: 3g; Sodium: 12mg

White Bean and Chickpea Hummus

5 INGREDIENT **30 MINUTES** **EASY PREP** **GLUTEN-FREE** **NO COOK** **NUT-FREE** **ONE POT** **SOY-FREE**

MAKES 3 CUPS PREP TIME: 5 minutes

I love a fast bean dip, and this one takes the cake. The combination of the creamy white beans with hummus's traditional chickpeas yields a wonderful texture without adding a high-fat component, like tahini or oil. Pair this with veggies or crackers, or use it as a sandwich spread or filling for Vegetable and Avocado Quesadillas (page 56).

1 (15-ounce) can
  chickpeas, drained
  and rinsed
1 (15-ounce) can white
  beans, drained
  and rinsed
3 tablespoons freshly
  squeezed lemon juice
2 teaspoons
  garlic powder
1 teaspoon onion powder

1. In a food processor or blender, combine the chickpeas, beans, lemon juice, garlic powder, and onion powder. Process for 1 to 2 minutes, or until the texture is smooth and creamy.

2. Serve right away or store in an airtight container in the refrigerator for up to 5 days.

VARIATION TIP: Add 1 teaspoon of chili powder and ½ teaspoon of cumin to create a chili hummus. Or toss in 1 teaspoon of smoked paprika and 1 tablespoon of maple syrup for a sweet and smoky hummus.

PER SERVING (¼ CUP): Calories: 61; Total fat: 1g; Total carbs: 11g; Fiber: 3g; Sugar: 1g; Protein: 3g; Sodium: 41mg

Carrot Cake Balls

30 MINUTES GLUTEN-FREE SOY-FREE

MAKES 24 BALLS PREP TIME: 10 minutes **COOK TIME:** 6 minutes

These are little bites of cake heaven. I love to have them in the refrigerator for an indulgent snack, as they more than satisfy my sweet tooth. I use peanut butter, but any nut or seed butter would work well.

2 cups unsweetened coconut flakes

1 carrot, coarsely chopped

2 cups rolled oats

½ cup smooth natural peanut butter

½ cup pure maple syrup

¼ cup coarsely chopped pecans

1 teaspoon ground cinnamon

½ teaspoon vanilla extract

½ teaspoon ground ginger

1. In a medium sauté pan or skillet over medium-high heat, toast the coconut, stirring or flipping occasionally, for 3 to 6 minutes, until lightly browned. Remove from the heat.

2. In a food processor, pulse the carrot until finely chopped but not pureed. Transfer the carrot to a small bowl and set aside.

3. In the food processor (it is okay if there is a little carrot in the bowl from the previous step), combine the toasted coconut flakes and oats. Pulse until coarsely ground but not so much that the ingredients become a flour.

4. Return the carrots to the processor and add the peanut butter, maple syrup, pecans, cinnamon, vanilla, and ginger. Pulse until the dough starts to form a ball.

5. Scoop out 2 tablespoons of dough and roll into a ball. Repeat with remaining dough. You should end up with about 24 balls.

6. Store in an airtight container in the refrigerator for up to 2 weeks.

INGREDIENT TIP: Desiccated coconut will work for this recipe, but the strands don't break down as well as flaked coconut.

PER SERVING (2 BALLS): Calories: 196; Total fat: 12g; Total carbs: 20g; Fiber: 3g; Sugar: 6g; Protein: 4g; Sodium: 10mg

Super Seed Chocolate Bark

GLUTEN-FREE SOY-FREE

PREP TIME: 10 minutes, plus 1 hour to chill **COOK TIME:** 20 minutes **SERVES:** 6

This snack is a candy that satisfies the plant-based way of eating. Who doesn't love a piece of chocolate every now and then? This bark mixes up quickly but takes about 1 hour to set in the refrigerator.

1 cup vegan dark
   chocolate
   chips, chunks, or
   chopped bars
¼ cup chopped unsalted
   pistachios
1 tablespoon
   sesame seeds
1 tablespoon raw hulled
   pumpkin seeds

1. Line a small baking sheet with parchment paper.

2. Fill the bottom of a double boiler or a medium saucepan with a few inches of water and bring to a boil over high heat. Lower the heat to medium to keep the water at a simmer. Place the chocolate in the top of the double boiler or in a heatproof bowl that fits over the saucepan (the bottom of the bowl should not touch the water) and place it over the simmering water. Using a silicone spatula, stir frequently until the chocolate has melted. Remove from the heat.

3. In a small bowl, combine the pistachios, sesame seeds, and pumpkin seeds.

4. Scrape the melted chocolate into the center of the prepared baking sheet and spread it into a layer about ¼ inch thick (the chocolate won't cover the entire pan). Sprinkle the nuts and seeds over the top. Refrigerate for at least 1 hour.

5. Break the chocolate bark into 10 rough pieces. Serve immediately or store in an airtight container at room temperature for up to 1 week or in the refrigerator for up to 2 weeks.

VARIATION TIP: For a fun topping option, crumble this over the Muesli and Yogurt Breakfast Parfait (page 29).

PER SERVING: Calories: 170; Total fat: 12g; Total carbs: 15g; Fiber: 2g; Sugar: 5g; Protein: 3g; Sodium: 8mg

Chickpea Cookie Dough

30 MINUTES · GLUTEN-FREE · SOY-FREE · NO COOK

PREP TIME: 20 minutes **SERVES:** 8

Chickpeas take center stage in this treat. You can feel good about eating cookie dough (finally!), since chickpeas are packed with protein. Enjoy your newfound craving with apple slices, celery stalks, or my preference, a spoon. Add some dried fruit or vegan chocolate chips to really knock it out of the park.

1 (15-ounce) can chickpeas, drained and rinsed

½ cup smooth natural peanut butter

2 tablespoons pure maple syrup

1½ teaspoons vanilla extract

½ teaspoon ground cinnamon

2 tablespoons pecans

1. Pour the chickpeas into a bowl and fill the bowl with water. Gently rub the chickpeas between your hands until you feel the skins coming off. Add more water to the bowl and let the skins float to the surface. Using your hand, scoop out the skins. Drain some of the water and repeat this step once more to remove as many of the chickpea skins as possible. Drain to remove all the water. Set the chickpeas aside.

2. In a food processor, combine the chickpeas, peanut butter, maple syrup, vanilla, and cinnamon. Process for 2 minutes. Scrape down the sides and process for 2 minutes more, or until the dough is smooth and the ingredients are evenly distributed.

3. Add the pecans and pulse to combine but not fully process.

4. Store in an airtight container in the refrigerator for up to 1 week.

PREPARATION TIP: Peeling the chickpeas before adding them to the food processor is an important step because it gives you a smooth cookie dough and takes away the chickpea flavor.

PER SERVING: Calories: 164; Total fat: 10g; Total carbs: 14g; Fiber: 3g; Sugar: 3g; Protein: 6g; Sodium: 64mg

Mini No-Bake Cheesecakes

FREEZES WELL GLUTEN-FREE NO COOK SOY-FREE

PREP TIME: 5 minutes, plus 6 hours to chill **SERVES:** 6

I love this sweet, tangy filling atop the graham cracker-inspired crust in these no-bake cheesecakes. I like to find unsweetened plant-based yogurt for this recipe that has the fewest ingredients. Kite Hill brand is my favorite. I have also tried it with sweetened plant-based vanilla yogurt and simply omitted the maple syrup and vanilla in the filling.

For the crust

½ cup pitted dates

½ cup rolled oats

¼ cup raw walnuts

2 tablespoons pure
  maple syrup

¼ teaspoon nutritional
  yeast

¼ teaspoon
  vanilla extract

½ teaspoon ground
  cinnamon

For the filling

1 cup raw cashews

1 cup unsweetened
  plant-based yogurt

2 tablespoons pure
  maple syrup

1 tablespoon freshly
  squeezed lemon juice

½ teaspoon
  vanilla extract

1. **Make the crust:** In a food processor, process the dates, oats, walnuts, maple syrup, nutritional yeast, vanilla, and cinnamon to a crumbly texture.

2. **Make the filling:** In a high-efficiency blender, blend the cashews, yogurt, maple syrup, lemon juice, and vanilla until smooth.

3. Line a 6-cup muffin tin with parchment paper cut to fit each cup. Spoon 2 tablespoons of the crust mixture into each cup and press down firmly with the back of the spoon or a measuring cup. Add 2 tablespoons of the filling to each cup.

4. Place in the freezer for up to 6 hours.

5. To serve, allow the cups to sit on the counter for 20 minutes until they soften slightly.

VARIATION TIP: These are delicious on their own, but you can also make a warm berry compote to top them by mixing 1 cup of fresh or frozen berries with ¼ cup of raisins and simmering until thickened, about 5 minutes.

PER SERVING: Calories: 290; Total fat: 15g; Total carbs: 35g; Fiber: 3g; Sugar: 19g; Protein: 8g; Sodium: 10mg

Chocolatey Mousse

5 INGREDIENT **GLUTEN-FREE** **NO COOK** **NUT-FREE**

PREP TIME: 10 minutes, plus 1 hour to chill **SERVES:** 6

Tofu can be a dinner or a dessert, and it does not disappoint in this protein-packed chocolatey mousse. I love to serve this with fresh berries and a few mint leaves for a fancy and flavorful treat.

1 (12-ounce) block firm
  tofu, drained
¼ cup pure maple syrup
¼ cup unsweetened
  cocoa powder
1 teaspoon vanilla extract
1 cup fresh berries
  (optional)
¼ cup fresh mint leaves
  (optional)

1. In a food processor, combine the tofu, maple syrup, cocoa powder, and vanilla extract and pulse until smooth and thick. Don't overprocess! Transfer to a bowl and refrigerate for at least 1 hour or up to overnight before serving.

2. Spoon the mousse into dessert bowls and serve topped with the berries (if using) and mint (if using).

INGREDIENT TIP: While I like a firm tofu, you can absolutely use shelf-stable silken tofu. The texture varies a bit, but it'll work just fine.

PER SERVING: Calories: 84; Total fat: 3g; Total carbs: 12g; Fiber: 2g; Sugar: 8g; Protein: 5g; Sodium: 15mg

5-Ingredient Chocolate Cookies

5 INGREDIENT **30 MINUTES** **EASY PREP** **GLUTEN-FREE** **SOY-FREE**

MAKES 12 COOKIES PREP TIME: 5 minutes **COOK TIME:** 15 minutes

I set out to make a chocolate cookie that is perfect for dunking in a mug of vegan hot cocoa or a bit of plant-based milk, and this is it! Rich and decadent, this cookie will satisfy any chocolate craving. I like to process oat flour myself; I simply add several cups to my high-efficiency blender and let it do the work. Then I store it in an airtight container until I am ready to use it.

1 cup oat flour

⅓ cup unsweetened cocoa powder

½ cup almond butter

¼ cup pure maple syrup

1 teaspoon vanilla extract

2 tablespoons water

1. Preheat the oven to 350° F and line a baking sheet with parchment paper.

2. In a large bowl, mix together the oat flour and cocoa powder until combined.

3. Add the almond butter, maple syrup, and vanilla and stir to combine using a rubber spatula or wooden spoon. If the dough is too dry or crumbly, add the water, 1 tablespoon at a time, and stir to combine.

4. Once the cookie dough is soft and has enough moisture to roll into a ball, scoop 1-tablespoon balls onto the baking sheet about 1 inch apart. Gently press the balls into flat cookies. Repeat until all the dough is used.

5. Bake for 10 to 12 minutes, until the cookies start to brown.

6. Remove from the oven and allow to cool for 10 minutes on the baking sheet before transferring to a wire rack to cool completely. Serve.

VARIATION TIP: To make a nut-free version, use a seed-based alternative, such as sunflower seed butter.

PER SERVING (2 COOKIES): Calories: 245; Total fat: 14g; Total carbs: 27g; Fiber: 5g; Sugar: 9g; Protein: 8g; Sodium: 10mg

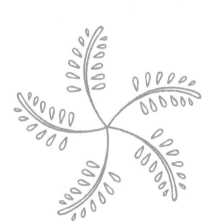

Mint Brownie Date Bars

5 INGREDIENT **30 MINUTES** **FREEZES WELL** **GLUTEN-FREE** **NO COOK** **NUT-FREE**
ONE POT **SOY-FREE**

PREP TIME: 10 minutes, plus 15 minutes to chill **SERVES:** 6

Chocolate and mint come together beautifully in these no-bake brownie bars. I like to keep these on hand in case of chocolate emergencies. They also work very well for holiday cookie trades and exchanges or as a refreshing, chocolatey treat in the heat of the summer.

1 cup pitted
  Medjool dates
1 cup rolled oats
2 tablespoons unsweet-
  ened cocoa powder
¼ teaspoon mint extract
¼ cup cacao nibs or
  vegan chocolate chips

1. Sort through the dates and ensure there are no pits.

2. In a food processor, combine the dates, oats, cocoa powder, mint extract, and cacao nibs. Pulse a few times to combine, scrape down the sides, and process until a ball forms. Shape the dough into a ½-inch-thick rectangle and cut it into six bars.

3. Stack the bars with a sheet of parchment paper or wax paper between them to avoid sticking. Refrigerate in a zip-top bag for up to 2 weeks, or freeze in an airtight container for 4 to 6 months.

INGREDIENT TIP: It is important to check dates for pits before processing because just one pit can damage your food processor blade or ruin a whole batch of bars.

PER SERVING: Calories: 189; Total fat: 4g; Total carbs: 37g; Fiber: 5g; Sugar: 13g; Protein: 3g; Sodium: 9mg

Berry Cobbler

GLUTEN-FREE NUT-FREE SOY-FREE

PREP TIME: 10 minutes **COOK TIME:** 30 minutes **SERVES:** 4

Warm, gooey, and topped with sweet oat biscuit-style topping, this easy dessert will become a new favorite. One time I made this with a delightful berry mix that had dark cherries in it, and it was bursting with flavor. If you can find a frozen cherry-berry mix, I highly recommend it.

1 (16-ounce) bag frozen
  mixed berries
¼ cup, plus 3 tablespoons
  pure maple syrup
1 tablespoon freshly
  squeezed lemon juice
½ teaspoon
  vanilla extract
1 tablespoon chia seeds
¼ teaspoon ground
  cinnamon
½ cup rolled oats
¾ cup oat flour
¼ cup unsweetened
  plant-based milk
1 tablespoon tahini

1. Preheat the oven to 350° F.

2. In an 8-by-8-inch baking dish, mix together the berries, ¼ cup of maple syrup, the lemon juice, vanilla, chia seeds, and cinnamon until well combined.

3. In a medium bowl, mix the oats, oat flour, milk, remaining 3 tablespoons of maple syrup, and the tahini until well combined.

4. Dollop the oat mixture atop the berry mixture and evenly spread it out.

5. Bake for 30 minutes, until the oat mixture starts to brown and the berry mixture is thickened and bubbling.

6. Let set for 3 to 5 minutes before serving, then enjoy!

INGREDIENT TIP: You can use fresh berries in this recipe as well.

PER SERVING: Calories: 557; Total fat: 12g; Total carbs: 111g; Fiber: 13g; Sugar: 54g; Protein: 13g; Sodium: 46mg

Cherry Nice Cream

5 INGREDIENT · 30 MINUTES · FREEZES WELL · GLUTEN-FREE · NO COOK · NUT-FREE · ONE POT · SOY-FREE

PREP TIME: 10 minutes · **SERVES:** 6

Nice Cream, made from frozen bananas, is perfect on a hot summer day or even when cozied up by the fire. I always have some banana chunks in my freezer; when the bananas get spotty and a little soft, I peel them, break them into pieces, and freeze them in a single layer on a baking sheet. Once they are frozen, I transfer them to a freezer-safe, airtight container so I can make this quick treat anytime. This cherry version is as pretty as it is delicious.

6 frozen bananas, cut into chunks (about 6 cups)

3 cups frozen pitted cherries

1. In a food processor, combine the bananas and cherries, and purée, scraping down the sides of the processor as needed, until smooth and creamy.

2. Serve immediately.

VARIATION TIP: Try frozen pineapple, blueberries, blackberries, or mango in place of the cherries.

PER SERVING: Calories: 152; Total fat: 1g; Total carbs: 39g; Fiber: 5g; Sugar: 21g; Protein: 2g; Sodium: 2mg

Strawberry-Watermelon Ice Pops

5 INGREDIENT   GLUTEN-FREE   FREEZES WELL   NO COOK   NUT-FREE   SOY-FREE

PREP TIME: 5 minutes, plus 6 hours to freeze   **SERVES:** 6

I love having these ice pops on hand for a chilled treat in the summer months. The combination of juicy fruits and tart lime juice is refreshing and bright. Be sure to use just the red part of the watermelon for the sweetest ice pop treats.

4 cups watermelon cubes

**4 strawberries,
    tops removed**

**2 tablespoons freshly
    squeezed lime juice**

1. In a blender, combine the watermelon, strawberries, and lime juice. Blend for 1 to 2 minutes, until well combined.

2. Pour evenly into six ice-pop molds, insert ice-pop sticks, and freeze for at least 6 hours before serving.

PREPARATION TIP: Silicon or stainless steel ice-pop molds can be purchased online or at some specialty grocery stores. Or you can always use paper cups!

PER SERVING: Calories: 38; Total fat: 0g; Total carbs: 10g; Fiber: 1g; Sugar: 7g; Protein: 1g; Sodium: 1mg

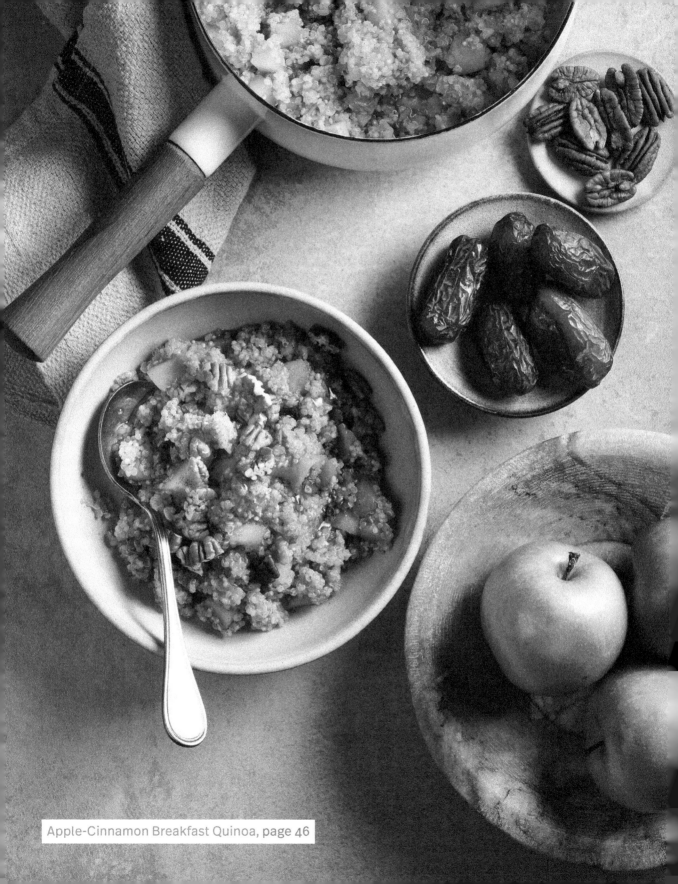

Apple-Cinnamon Breakfast Quinoa, page 46

Cooking Basics Chart

A healthy plant-based diet is built around whole-food ingredients such as rice, grains, beans, and starchy vegetables. These can be cooked in many ways using common kitchen tools and appliances. By finding your favorite ways to regularly prepare starchy staples, you can have healthy, ready-to-warm foods always available.

	METHOD	RATIO OF STAPLE TO WATER	SETTING AND COOK TIME	YIELD (FOR 1 CUP DRY STAPLE)
Brown rice	Stovetop	1:2	Bring to boil, then simmer, covered, for 30 minutes	2 cups
	Pressure cooker	1:1 ¼	Manual for 15 minutes	
	Slow cooker	1:1 ½	High for 2 ½ hours Low for 5 hours	
Quinoa	Stovetop	1:1 ½	Bring to boil, then simmer, covered, for 20 minutes	3 cups
	Pressure cooker	1:1	Manual for 1 minute	
	Slow cooker	1:1 ½	High for 2 ½ hours Low for 5 hours	

![grain icon]	METHOD	RATIO OF STAPLE TO WATER	SETTING AND COOK TIME	YIELD (FOR 1 CUP DRY STAPLE)
Potato, whole (e.g., red, white, yellow)	Oven	—	400°F for 40 to 50 minutes	N/A
	Stovetop	Water to cover all potatoes	Boil, covered, for 20 to 30 minutes	
	Pressure cooker	1 cup water	Manual for 10 to 15 minutes	
	Slow cooker	1 to 2 tablespoons water	High for 2 to 3 hours Low for 4 to 6 hours	
Sweet potato, whole	Oven	—	400°F for 40 to 50 minutes	N/A
	Stovetop	Water to cover all sweet potatoes	Boil for 20 to 30 minutes	
	Pressure cooker	1 cup water	Manual for 15 to 20 minutes	
	Slow cooker	1 to 2 tablespoons water	High for 4 hours Low for 6 hours	

	METHOD	RATIO OF STAPLE TO WATER	SETTING AND COOK TIME	YIELD (FOR 1 CUP DRY STAPLE)
Beans*	Stovetop	1:3	Soak overnight, then bring to boil and simmer for 45 to 60 minutes	2¼ cups
	Pressure cooker	1:3	Dry: Manual for 25 to 30 minutes Soaked: Manual for 8 to 10 minutes	
	Slow cooker	1:3	Soak overnight, then cook on High for 3 to 4 hours or Low for 6 to 8 hours	
Lentils	Stovetop	1:3	Bring to boil, reduce heat, and simmer for 25 minutes	2½ cups
	Pressure cooker	1:3	Dry: Manual for 10 minutes Soaked: N/A	
	Slow cooker	1:3	High for 3 to 4 hours Low for 6 to 8 hours	

*You can use 1½ cups of cooked beans and ½ cup of cooking liquid wherever beans are called for (1½ cups of drained and rinsed beans, if recipe indicates).

	METHOD	RATIO OF STAPLE TO WATER	SETTING AND COOK TIME	YIELD (FOR 1 CUP DRY STAPLE)
Chick-peas	Stovetop	1:3	Soak overnight, bring to boil, and simmer for 35 to 40 minutes	2½ to 3 cups
	Pressure cooker	1:3	Dry: Manual for 35 to 40 minutes Soaked: Manual for 10 to 15 minutes	
	Slow cooker	1:3	Soak overnight, then cook on High for 3 to 4 hours or Low for 6 to 8 hours	
Squash, diced (e.g., acorn, butter-nut, kabocha)	Oven	—	Bake on parchment paper-lined baking sheet for 25 to 30 minutes at 400°F	N/A
	Stovetop	Water to cover all squash	Boil, covered, for 10 to 15 minutes	
	Pressure cooker	1 cup water	Manual for 5 minutes	
	Slow cooker	1 to 2 tablespoons water	High for 3 hours Low for 6 hours	

Measurement Conversions

Volume Equivalents (Liquid)

US STANDARD	US STANDARD (OUNCES)	METRIC (APPROXIMATE)
2 tablespoons	1 fl. oz.	30 mL
¼ cup	2 fl. oz.	60 mL
½ cup	4 fl. oz.	120 mL
1 cup	8 fl. oz.	240 mL
1½ cups	12 fl. oz.	355 mL
2 cups or 1 pint	16 fl. oz.	475 mL
4 cups or 1 quart	32 fl. oz.	1 L
1 gallon	128 fl. oz.	4 L

Oven Temperatures

FAHRENHEIT	CELSIUS (APPROXIMATE)
250°F	120°C
300°F	150°C
325°F	165°C
350°F	180°C
375°F	190°C
400°F	200°C
425°F	220°C
450°F	230°C

Volume Equivalents (Dry)

US STANDARD	METRIC (APPROXIMATE)
⅛ teaspoon	0.5 mL
¼ teaspoon	1 mL
½ teaspoon	2 mL
¾ teaspoon	4 mL
1 teaspoon	5 mL
1 tablespoon	15 mL
¼ cup	59 mL
⅓ cup	79 mL
½ cup	118 mL
⅔ cup	156 mL
¾ cup	177 mL
1 cup	235 mL
2 cups or 1 pint	475 mL
3 cups	700 mL
4 cups or 1 quart	1 L

Weight Equivalents

US STANDARD	METRIC (APPROXIMATE)
½ ounce	15 g
1 ounce	30 g
2 ounces	60 g
4 ounces	115 g
8 ounces	225 g
12 ounces	340 g
16 ounces or 1 pound	455 g

Index

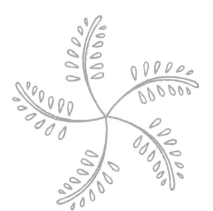

Acknowledgments

I first want to take a moment to thank the fans of VegInspired. Your ongoing support and engagement fuel my continued work in the plant-based community.

Included in those fans is my biggest fan—my husband, John. You always know just what to say to inspire me to get into the kitchen and create another fabulous dish or meal. Thank you; your support and feedback have made me a better chef.

I want to acknowledge the plant-based enthusiasts, doctors, and researchers in this arena who have inspired me throughout my plant-based journey. Your work changed my life.

To my family and friends who checked in on me during the writing of this book, thank you.

To the team at Callisto Media, again you have managed to make my words and recipes jump off the page as timeless inspiration. Thank you!

To my readers, I hope this book inspires you to give a new plant-based recipe a try.

About the Author

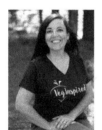

Kathy A. Davis is a cookbook author, plant-based lifestyle coach, and founder of VegInspired.com. She has been creating delicious plant-based recipes for more than six years. Kathy is also the author of the *30-Minute Whole-Food, Plant-Based Cookbook*.

Kathy is passionate about a plant-based lifestyle with healthy recipes, and loves sharing her passion through her unique plant-based lifestyle coaching program. She is currently traveling the United States in a fifth-wheel camper with her husband, John, and their three cats. Together they have a goal to visit all of the US national parks.

CPSIA information can be obtained
at www.ICGtesting.com
Printed in the USA
JSHW051113230521
15039JS00001B/2

9 781648 769405